Public Health:
Social Context and Action

Public Health: Social Context and Action

Edited by
Angela Scriven
Sebastian Garman

 Open University Press

Open University Press
McGraw-Hill Education
McGraw-Hill House
Shoppenhangers Road
Maidenhead
Berkshire
England
SL6 2QL

email: enquiries@openup.co.uk
world wide web: www.openup.co.uk

and Two Penn Plaza, New York, NY 10121–2289, USA

First published 2007

A catalogue record for this book is available from the British Library.

ISBN 13: 9780335221509 (pb) 9780335221516 (hb)
ISBN 10: 0335221509 (pb) 0335221513 (hb)

Library of Congress Cataloguing-in-Publication Data
CIP data applied for

Typeset by YHT Ltd, London
Printed in Poland by OZ Graf. S.A.
www.polskabook.pl

The McGraw·Hill Companies

Contents

Part 2: Public health action

Notes on contributors

Amanda Amos is Professor of Health Promotion in the Division of Community Health Sciences at Edinburgh University. She has been teaching and researching health promotion for over 20 years. Her research has focused on a range of smoking issues from the individual to community and societal levels. She is a member of the Boards of ASH Scotland, the European Network for Smoking Prevention and the International Network of Women Against Tobacco (Europe); a senior editor of the international journal *Tobacco Control*; and Chair of the researchers' group of the Scottish Tobacco Control Alliance.

Mel Bartley is Professor of Medical Sociology in the Department of Epidemiology and Public Health, University College London. Her main areas of research are those that cross the boundaries between sociology and epidemiology, including gender differences in health, health inequalities, the relationship between health, work and unemployment, and resilience in the life course. Mel also has an interest in the history of occupational health and the relationship between research and policy. She has published widely in these areas, and also written two books, *Authorities and Partisans: The Debate on Unemployment and Health* (Edinburgh University Press 1982) and *Health Inequality: An Introduction to Concepts, Theories and Methods* (Polity Press 2003), and co-edited the Sociology and Health and Illness monograph *The Sociology of Health Inequalities* (Blackwell 1998).

Linda Bauld is a Reader in Social Policy at the University of Bath. She is an applied policy researcher with a particular interest in public health policy. Most of her recent work has involved the evaluation of complex community based interventions to improve health. Along with the evaluation of several national programmes, including Health Action Zones in England, she has been involved with a number of studies examining the efficacy of public health interventions, most notably smoking cessation services in Scotland and England. She has published several books and articles in a range of peer reviewed journals.

Hannah Bradby is Co-director of the Institute of Health at the University of Warwick where she teaches in the Medical School and the Department of Sociology. Her publications in the field of ethnicity and health include a paper, 'Watch out for the aunties: young British Asians' accounts of identity and substance use', forthcoming in the journal *Sociology of Health and Illness*, and a fictionalised account of her ethnographic research, *Skinfull*, published by Onlywomen Press.

Tarani Chandola is a senior lecturer in Medical Sociology in the Department of Epidemiology and Public Health, University College London. He works on the Whitehall II study and other longitudinal datasets. He obtained a DPhil in sociology from Nuffield College, University of Oxford in 1998. His work includes research on the measurement of social position in relation to health, explaining social, ethnic and geographical variations in health and analysing the role of psychosocial factors in explaining social inequalities in health. Dr Chandola is one of the course organizers on the UCL MSc Health and Society: Social Epidemiology course.

Jeff Collin is a lecturer in the Centre for International Public Health Policy, University of Edinburgh. A political scientist by background, he was previously based at the London School of Hygiene and Tropical Medicine and his research currently focuses on globalization and tobacco control. Using corporate documents disclosed following litigation, this work analyses attempts by transnational tobacco companies to influence public policy, particularly in developing countries. Additional research interests include developments in global health governance and the health impacts of population mobility and trade liberalization.

Paul Fleming is Associate Dean of the Faculty of Life and Health Sciences at the University of Ulster, where he established and has taught on the MSc in Health Promotion since 1992. A health promotion specialist and post-primary school teacher by background, he has held a variety of posts in health promotion and teaching over the last 30 years. His current research interests include health promoting settings, particularly the workplace and also sexual health. He has co-authored a book, *Impacting Health at Work*, has published extensively in peer reviewed journals and is editor of the *Journal of Environmental Health Research*.

Colin Fudge is Professor of Urban Environment and Pro Vice-Chancellor at UWE, Bristol. He has held senior positions in government and academia in the UK, Sweden, Australia and the EU, was awarded an Honorary Fellowship of the Royal Institute of British Architects for his work on urban sustainability, and the title of Royal Professor by the Swedish Academy of Sciences. He is chair of the EU Expert Group on the Urban Environment, founding director of the WHO Collaborative Research Centre on Healthy Cities and Urban Policy, visiting professor, Italy and Sweden, and a board member at Chalmers University. He has written more than 80 articles and reports, ten books, numerous book chapters and presented more than 100 conference papers.

Sebastian Garman is Senior Tutor to the School of Health Sciences and Social Care at Brunel University in London. He is course leader for the MSc in Health Promotion and Public Health. He has helped design, teach and publish for health-related courses for 30 years, including joint editorship of the book *Promoting Health: Global Perspectives* (Palgrave Macmillan 2005). He is a sociologist with a research interest in collective memory and identity. He is on the Advisory Council of the Association for the Study of Ethnicity and Nationalism and on the editorial committee of its journal, *Nations and Nationalism*.

Ben Gidley is a research fellow at the Centre for Urban and Community Research, which is attached to the sociology department at Goldsmiths College, London. He has worked on a variety of research projects, mainly in London, around issues of youth, ethnicity, migration, social exclusion and community development. In particular, he has led a number of evaluations of local social policy interventions, such as Sure Start, Single Regeneration Budget programmes and neighbourhood renewal projects.

Jenny Head is Senior Lecturer in Statistics in the Department of Epidemiology and Public Health, University College London. Having previously worked on large-scale studies such as the National Child Development Study she coordinates the Medical and Social Statistics group, a network of statisticians working in the department. She is a member of the Whitehall II study management team and also a co-investigator on a component project of the ESRC priority network on capability and resilience. She is principal investigator on a project investigating the health impacts of work-related stress funded by the Health and Safety Executive.

David Hunter is Professor of Health Policy and Management at Durham University. He is Director of the Centre for Public Policy and Health in the School for Health located at the Wolfson Research Institute. A political scientist by background, he has researched and published widely in the field of health policy and management for nearly 30 years. Among his books are *Desperately Seeking Solutions: Rationing Health Care* (Longman 1997) and *Public Health Policy* (Polity 2003). He is co-editor with Sian Griffiths of *New Perspectives in Public Health* (2nd edn, Radcliffe 2006). He is Chair of the UK Public Health Association and a member of NICE's R&D Scientific Advisory Group.

Martin King is a Principal Lecturer in the Division of Psychology and Social Change at Manchester Metropolitan University. He has worked in the field of health promotion and public health in both the NHS and local authority settings. He is co-editor of *Representing Health: Discourses of Health and Illness in the Media* (Palgrave Macmillan 2005). He is currently completing his PhD on *Representations of Masculinity in the Mass Media 1960– 1970* and is a regular columnist for the *Journal of the Royal Society for the Promotion of Health*.

Roderick Lawrence is Professor at the Faculty of Economic and Social Sciences at the University of Geneva. He has served as a consultant to the Organization for Economic Cooperation and Development, the Economic Commission for Europe and the World Health Organization. From 1998 to 2003 he was Chairperson of the Evaluation Advisory Committee of the WHO-EURO Healthy Cities project.

Kelley Lee is Reader in Global Health at the London School of Hygiene and Tropical Medicine. She has chaired the WHO Scientific Resource Group on Globalization, Trade and Health. Her research focuses on the global dimensions of communicable and non-communicable diseases, and the implications arising for global governance. Current projects include analysis of tobacco industry documents, and the links between health, foreign policy and security. Her books include *Health Impacts of Globalization* (Palgrave Macmillan 2003), *Globalization and Health: An Introduction* (Palgrave Macmillan 2003) and *Global Change and Health* (Open University Press 2005).

Yaojun Li is a Reader in Sociological Analysis at Birmingham University. His research interests are in social mobility and social stratification, social capital, political preferences, occupational and educational attainment and religious identity. He has published widely in these areas. His papers have appeared in many leading sociology journals such as the *European Sociological Review*, *British Journal of Sociology*, *Sociology*, *Work, Employment and Society*, *Sociological Review*, *Explorations in Sociology*, *Sociological Research*, *Sociological Research Online* and *Ageing and Society*. He has also conducted numerous projects for the ESRC and other government bodies such as the DTI and the National Assembly of Wales.

Mhairi Mackenzie is a Senior Lecturer in Health Policy in the Department of Urban Studies at the University of Glasgow. She has been involved in the evaluation of a range of public health policy initiatives including Health Action Zones (where she managed the evaluation module focusing on whole systems change) and the National Health Demonstration Projects in Scotland. She has a particular interest in the evaluation of complex policy initiatives and the role of evidence in policy making.

Alex Marsh is Reader in Public Policy at the University of Bristol. His research has engaged with many aspects of the relationship between housing, the economy and society. Work on housing, health and care includes a study of the impact of housing on health using the National Child Development Study, an evaluation of innovative initiatives crossing the housing and care divide, and a review of the Disabled Facilities Grant. He has published widely, including co-editing *Housing and Public Policy* (Open 1998), *Homelessness* (The Policy Press 1999), and *Two Steps Forward: Housing Policy into the New Millennium* (The Policy Press 2001). He is currently a visiting academic consultant to the Law Commission, working on the reform of the structures to regulate private rented housing.

Antony Morgan is an Associate Director in the Centre for Public Health Excellence at the National Institute of Health and Clinical Excellence. His research interests include methodological issues relating to evidence based public health, promoting an assets-based approach to young people's health and development, and social approaches to tackling health inequalities.

Jennie Popay is Professor of Sociology and Public Health at the Institute for Health Research at Lancaster University. Her research interests include social and gender inequalities in health, the sociology of knowledge, the evaluation of complex social interventions and evidence synthesis. She is a co-convenor of the Qualitative Research Methods Group within the Cochrane Collaboration.

Graham Scambler is Professor of Medical Sociology at University College London. His interests range from issues of health and illness to social theory and the sociology of sport. He was Visiting Professor of Sociology at Emory University, Atlanta, USA, in 1998. He is founding co-editor of the international journal *Social Theory and Health*, which first appeared in 2003. His research areas include chronic illness and stigma, health inequalities and health issues in the sex industry. Recent books include: *Habermas, Critical*

Theory and Health (Routledge 2001); *Health and Social Change: A Critical Theory* (Open University Press 2002); *Sociology as Applied to Medicine* (5th edn, Saunders 2003); *Sport and Society: History, Power and Culture* (Open University Press 2005); and *Medical Sociology* (4 vols) (Routledge 2005).

Sasha Scambler is Lecturer in Sociology as Applied to Dentistry at King's College London. Her interests range from ageing and social participation in later life to chronic illness, disability and social theory. Research areas include children with profound multiple disability, barriers to oral healthcare for older people, and loneliness in later life. She has co-authored two chapters and has published in a number of peer reviewed journals.

Angela Scriven is Reader in Health Promotion at Brunel University, London. She has been teaching and researching in the field of health promotion for over 20 years and has published widely including the following edited books: *Health Promotion Alliances: Theory and Practice* (Palgrave Macmillan 1998), *Health Promotion: Professional Perspectives* (2nd edn, Palgrave Macmillan 2001), *Promoting Health: Global Perspectives* (Palgrave Macmillan 2005) and *Health Promoting Practice: The Contribution of Nurses and Allied Health Professionals* (Palgrave Macmillan 2005). Her research is centred on the relationship between health promotion policy and practice within specific contexts.

Nick Watson is Professor of Disability Studies and Director of Strathclyde Centre for Disability Research at the University of Glasgow. He has written widely on a range of disability issues including disabled children, disability and identity, theorizing disability and the role of impairment, care and personal support, and disability and politics. He has co-edited a number of collections, including *Disability and Culture* (Pearson 2003) and *Reframing the Body* (Palgrave 2001).

Acknowledgements

We would like to acknowledge and thank all the authors for their enthusiasm and support of this text and the many people who have assisted the contributors with the development of ideas in individual chapters. A special word of thanks goes to Bethan Rylance for her highly efficient support and assistance in finalizing the manuscript and to Rachel Gear from the Open University Press for her encouragement throughout. The Economic and Social Research Council funded the research on which both Chapters 5 and 6 were based, and the Data Archive made available the British Household Panel Survey data for analysis in Chapter 6.

Foreword

As we move into the early years of the twenty-first century, it is increasingly clear that public health is coming of age. There is now growing recognition among political decision-makers that measures to promote and protect health require more than exhortations to change health-damaging behaviour. Health is determined by the conditions in which we live out our everyday lives. Our social and economic circumstances, physical environment and global interactions interplay with our genetic make-up and learned behaviours to create or damage our potential for health and happiness. Improving public health is therefore a multisectoral, multidisciplinary endeavour, requiring all sectors to play a part. Moreover, the dividend arising from better health will also be felt by all sections of society. Poor health results in social and financial costs. Good health is an economic resource.

But the challenges are also enormous. The sometimes insidious impact of the mass media, combined with the effect of health-damaging products marketed in the interests of corporate profit, constrain the possibilities for health improvement. New and re-emerging communicable diseases, coupled with ever more efficient vectors for global transmission, threaten both developed and developing nations. To these challenges, we must also add the consequences of natural and man-made disasters. The effects of climate change, inadequate environmental planning and the ever growing threat of terrorism have all ascended the public health agenda.

In addition, we have seen growing disparities between social groups. Inequalities in health and wealth are growing not just between nations, but within them. Cultural and ethnic differences, social exclusion and differential access to the fundamental determinants of health, such as education, housing and economic resources, are all playing a role in the marginalization of certain groups in society. The need for effective public health interventions has never been greater.

This book helps readers navigate through the complexity of factors that impinge upon our health and wellbeing. The early chapters consider the impact of socioeconomic influences upon both individual and population health. In so doing, they take account of the particular circumstances associated with marginalized and minority groups. That health and ill health demonstrate a clear social gradient is well known. This anthology explores the evidence and draws out some of the implications for public health practice. Although most public health practitioners tend to define communities by the health problems they face, this book also highlights the importance of social capital. Every population has its strengths as well as its weaknesses. Social organization, informal communication networks, civic participation, community leadership and local knowledge are all assets for health. Public health programmes must increasingly map these assets as the starting point for action as well as identify the health challenges.

It is well known that the mass media exert an enormous influence over public perceptions, attitudes and behaviours. If this were not the case, commercial enterprises would not invest huge sums of money in media driven marketing and advertising campaigns. In considering the use of media strategies to promote health, however, it is questionable whether the public health agencies have the wherewithal or resources to exploit the full potential of mass communication technologies.

The public health community has sometimes been accused of too much analysis and too little action. Later chapters explore the translation of theory and evidence into practical application. Effective intervention demands the right policies, principles, processes and partnerships. Politicians and other decision makers are coming to understand that the comprehensive, contemporary threats to health require an equally comprehensive approach. It is no longer viewed as realistic to think that public education alone can bring about a radical transformation in our health prospects. The full range of policy instruments and opportunities available to our political leaders must be deployed if we are to meet the challenges of the new millennium.

Health is now well understood to be a function, at least in part, of the settings in which we work, live and play. The past 25 years have seen a growing emphasis on schools, workplaces and local neighbourhoods as the focus for public health action – perhaps not surprisingly, as they help define the physical and social world in which we act out our daily lives. They offer a manageable environment for working with specific communities.

It is also essential to address the underpinning social, economic and educational determinants of health, alongside the settings approach. In so doing, we shall be simultaneously tackling not just one or two health issues, but many. Drawing on the practical expertise and knowledge of the authors, this book embeds current thinking in contemporary practice. From Sure Start to healthy workplaces, Health Action Zones to community regeneration, this volume makes the leap from research to action.

Professor Richard Parish FFPH, FRSH, FRIPH
Chief Executive
Royal Society of Health

1 Public health: an overview of social context and action

Angela Scriven

There has been a slow evolution in the concept of public health. As a field of activity it has shifted emphasis from being predominantly concerned with prevention of communicable diseases to include a much broader agenda and a multidisciplinary focus that includes the prevention of chronic disease. This evolutionary process has reached an important moment, with significant developments happening towards the end of the twentieth century that have given a new momentum to twenty-first-century public health. Of particular note has been the increased emphasis on the contribution of individual behaviour and lifestyles to disease, with public health programmes and strategies taking a population as well as an individual approach. The sociopolitical critiques surrounding these approaches have resulted in increased research and a greater understanding of the socioeconomic, environmental and cultural influences on behaviour and on health status. This text will add to this emergent body of knowledge, by examining a number of important debates around the social context of health, including the socioeconomic, environmental and cultural elements. In addition to theoretical discourse, examples are provided of upstream and downstream strategies that have recently been introduced to tackle the social determinants of health. This combination of theory and praxis is essential in documenting thinking, frameworks and processes that are actively shaping public health today.

The two parts that make up the book have a discrete focus and a synergistic relationship. Part 1 centres on an analysis of the social context of health. Part 2 explores a number of public health actions that are designed specifically to address important issues identified in Part 1. There is cross referencing between both sections to establish clear links between theory and praxis. The idea is to locate social context theoretical debates and problems and then analyse the practical public health strategies and solutions that have been developed to address these. In doing this, there is much that is challenging, provocative and analytic not only of the social context in which public health takes place, but also of a range of public health actions.

Part 1 examines the social context in which public health policy is made and strategies are planned. The focus is on the assumptions, concepts and issues that shape the decision to act as well as the effectiveness of action. Part 2 presents a critical examination of strategic public health initiatives, in terms of their effectiveness and also in terms of wider considerations of evidence based practice. The theoretical issues will have international applicability. The discussion of public health policy and practice, however, will focus mainly on the UK environment, with authors drawing on international examples and comparisons where applicable and appropriate. Of note are the references made to relevant and recent public health research, policies and evidence based practice. In order for the text to have international relevance, ideas and issues are linked to national (including Scotland, Wales and Northern Ireland) and, where relevant, international health and public health policies and strategies. Future orientation includes an identification of trends, and the case for establishing new public health agendas and strategies is argued.

The second chapter in this introductory section offers both a detailed examination of the historical context of public health and an overview of the current agenda. Public health has a long history during which diverse ideological, disciplinary and social influences have shaped agendas and strategies. This chapter plots some of this history in the UK, with reference made where appropriate to US and European experience, and explores the new public health that dominates current policy and practice in the UK and beyond.

The social context of public health

The purpose of the first part of the book is to examine a range of issues relating to the social context of public health. It begins with a chapter outlining the social, political and economic environment and locates the changing social context in which public health decisions are made. It reviews social trends, including a focus on gender, and patterns of late modernity and the links made between these and health trends. Using national and international comparisons, and by drawing upon the discussion of the epidemiological transition, the food transition and demographic changes, examining age as a specific demographic issue, it explores the consequences of these changes for public health both in post industrial societies as well as in the emerging economies. The chapter ends with an analysis of the changing political institutions within which public health must operate, including those of family and marriage.

An examination of social patterning of health behaviours forms the focus of Chapter 4. Although the links between economic deprivation and ill health have been noted for as long as systematic records have been kept, the dynamic that maintains the link has been much disputed. Interesting recent evidence has given new impetus to the suggestion that the psychosocial dynamics of deprivation and inequality are as significant for health as the material factors themselves. Drawing on national and international data, and using examples at both a macro level, such as class and occupation, and a micro level, such as family, neighbourhood or schooling, this chapter reviews the evidence. A strong case is developed for the continuing importance of social class, and the implications for public health practice, both nationally and internationally, are identified.

Resilience and change is the context of Chapter 5, looking particularly at the relationship of work to health. The importance of work for the health of men and women has long been acknowledged in terms of the status, esteem, reciprocation, social support and material advantages it offers. Moreover, in the last decade important new evidence established the additional health costs of unemployment and even the threat of unemployment. By utilizing the concept of resilience, and by paying particular attention to gender, this chapter reassesses the evidence as well as reviewing research on the importance of the workplace, including workplace culture, to health. There is an examination of the claims that the present era of global change has added to insecurities and demands in the workplace that are jeopardizing improvements made to workplace health. The evidence for claims made about the significance of the work–life balance is also reviewed.

Social capital and social exclusion are dominant themes in the current public health agenda, and Chapter 6 gives this particular attention. The interrelationship between social exclusion, social capital and welfare has been much debated in recent years despite the limited amount of data on trends in the UK, and has been used to justify strategies for public health action. There has been a shortage of sustained analysis of the aetiology to show whether participation and trust breaks down social divisions or under some circumstances might even increase them. This chapter utilizes important new UK research to re-examine the assumptions behind the use of these concepts. There is a detailed exploration of the effects of sociocultural factors on civic participation and whether such links imply benefits for health in the UK and internationally.

Relating to both social capital and the politics of health are issues around ethnicity, which is the focus of the Chapter 7. Used in inconsistent and contradictory ways, the ideas of race and ethnicity have had an unfortunate relationship with public health research, sometimes problematizing ethnic categories rather than the focusing on improving health. Moreover, due to the aberrations of the history of the UK, ethnic health data on the English, Welsh and the Scots have not been focused on in the same way as data for Irish and other ethnic categories.

Chapter 8 continues with these themes by exploring disability, health, resistance and identity. With its particular adaptation of the social model of health, the disability movement in conjunction with gay pride, mental health survivors and feminist groups can make claims to have transformed approaches to public health action and research. This chapter examines present trends and prospects among disability groups that have shown some success in dismantling barriers of discrimination and prejudice as well as assessing contemporary strategies of engagement. By focusing on the UK, and by making international comparisons where appropriate, the manner in which groups are attempting to defend and extend health benefits gained through advocacy and the consolidation of networks of support is critically assessed.

Digital technologies have extended the power of mass communications at a time when ageing population structures, epidemiological changes, the food transition and lifestyle changes are focusing public health action towards advocacy and behaviour change. There is widespread acknowledgement that public health agencies are neither sophisticated in their management of mass communications nor knowledgeable about the effects of the mass media on health behaviours. Chapter 9, on mass media, lifestyle and public health, reviews the evidence, focusing on health and lifestyle issues, and advances the argument that the mass media, in particular television, present public health topics as a way of engaging prime-time viewers. There is an examination of the way programmers in the UK are capitalizing on public interest in health and lifestyle issues, using popular contemporary media formats in a way in which public health agencies seem unable or unwilling to emulate.

Globalization is a significant issue in public health policy and forms the focal point for Chapter 10, the final contribution to Part 1 of the book. Economic globalization has stimulated the formation of new institutions, networks and alliances in the management of public health. Using the cases of tobacco and population mobility as a focus for analysis, the changing international context and the manner in which globalization is transforming the institutions, policy and choices for public health in the UK is addressed. From public-private partnerships to long-term care, internationally negotiated global changes have major implications for public health. These dynamics are explored and the implications for the future of public health debated.

Public health action

Part 2, with its focus on public health action, begins with a detailed consideration of one aspect of action, healthy public policies, and examines whether these are just rhetoric or a reality. There is a detailed exploration of both the term and the concept of healthy public policies, as compared to public health policy, its roots and links to the social context of health and to public health promotion strategies, including World Health Organization (WHO) declarations. Developing healthy public policies involves alliances and partnerships that cross sector boundaries of traditional public policy making and foster a better interaction between personal, social and political arenas. International examples are used to compare with the UK situation, and to explore the extent and effectiveness of healthy public policies in terms of public health targets. Of particular note is the healthy public policy framework used in the Calgary health region in Canada. This is developed into a model that can be employed for the formation of healthy public policies at a local level.

Multidisciplinary action to address inequalities in health in the form of Health Action Zones (HAZs) is a practical example of healthy public policies in action. HAZs are multi-agency partnerships between the National Health Service (NHS), local authorities, including social services, the voluntary and business sectors and local communities. Their aim is to tackle inequalities in health in the most deprived areas of the country through health and social care modernization programmes. As well as tackling key priorities such as coronary health disease (CHD), cancer, mental health and issues such as teenage pregnancy, drug misuse prevention in vulnerable people, and smoking cessation, they are addressing other interdependent and wider determinants of health, such as housing, education and employment, and linking with other initiatives. HAZs also act as models for new ways of working and integrating these services and approaches into mainstream activity. Launched by the government in 1997, the HAZ initiative has focused on ways of tackling health inequalities in some of the most deprived areas in England. The Department of Health (DoH) agreed funding for HAZ until 2006. Chapter 12 examines the success of the initiative in tackling the social context determinants of health outlined in Part 1 of the book and concludes with a consideration of whether the initiative offers lessons for international public health practice.

Sure Start is the UK government's programme to deliver the best start in life for every child through multisector action that involves early education, childcare, health and family support. Chapter 13, on Sure Start, begins with a discussion of the principles underpinning the Sure Start initiative, the international precedents that might have helped inspire it, and the broader government strategies that shape it. The second part reports a selection of findings from a series of evaluations, including findings from the studies on the health impact of Sure Start on outcomes for children and parents, and findings on the involvement of different sorts of carers and families in Sure Start programmes. Conclusions are drawn as to whether the Sure Start initiative reflects an upstream approach to tackling inequalities in health and has international as well as national applicability.

Chapter 14 examines the emerging evidence around involving the public in attempts to improve and regenerate neighbourhoods and communities, both in the UK and internationally. The practical manifestation of regeneration public health is in partnerships and participation and its philosophical basis lies in empowerment. Evidence suggests, however, that public involvement does not always work very well in practice and that key decisions are taken by people outside the neighbourhoods or communities affected and are on the basis of health as an economic asset. The current position of the neighbourhood renewal approach to public health both within and outside the UK is critically explored, offering the Social Action for Health example of how cross-sector participative interventions aim to increase social inclusion and social capital, reduce inequalities and social exclusion, and empower neighbourhoods to take control of their own destinies.

The workplace has been identified as a key setting through which to improve health and reduce health inequalities. The Healthy Workplace initiative encapsulates a new approach to the problems of health at work. Chapter 15 examines what constitutes a healthy workplace and considers in detail the WHO's healthy workplace initiatives, citing examples of good practice at a UK and international level. The philosophy underpinning the initiative and the precise nature of healthy workplaces is examined and an assessment made of the benefits it affords to achieving public health targets and confronting the social determinants of health. Links with the wider picture of joined-up government are explored alongside a critique of partnership approaches, with business, trades unions and other organizations at international, national and local level.

Healthy cities, their context and relevance for urban health are the focus of Chapter 16. The health of people living in towns and cities is strongly determined by their living and working conditions, the quality of their physical and socioeconomic environment and the quality and accessibility of care services. This chapter discusses how the WHO Healthy Cities approach can offer comprehensive policy and planning solutions to urban health problems. There is a critical explanation of how Healthy Cities engages local governments in health development, through a process of political commitment, institutional changes, capacity-building, partnerships and other actions. National and international examples are used to demonstrate that urban poverty, the needs of vulnerable groups, the social, economic and environmental root causes of ill health and the positioning of health considerations in the centre of economic regeneration and urban development efforts are potential outcomes of Healthy Cities initiatives. The Belfast Declaration containing the principles and the goals of the 2003–7 phase of WHO Healthy Cities in Europe is outlined.

The social impact of anti-smoking public health action, particularly legislative action, forms the basis of the next chapter. There are numerous policy documents that set out the UK government policy to tackle tobacco use in Britain. The White Paper *Smoking*

Kills advocates a comprehensive range of measures each of which is intended to reduce smoking prevalence. It includes banning tobacco advertising, use of taxation, support for smokers wanting to quit, smoke free policies and a range of targets. The NHS Cancer Plan recognizes smoking to be a major contributor to prevalence of the disease and establishes prevention targets for reducing tobacco use in disadvantaged groups. There are non-binding policy statements from the European Council to the member states of the European Union (EU), covering issues that are not regulated at EU level, including retailing, vending machines, passive smoking, indirect advertising and disclosure of marketing budgets. The social context of smoking is considered and the impacts of some public health action designed to control tobacco use, both in the UK and abroad, are examined.

The final chapter of the book focuses on housing and explores the health and wellbeing aspects that make housing a public health action priority. Poor housing conditions are associated with a wide range of physical health conditions, including respiratory infections, asthma, lead poisoning and accidental injuries. What is less clear is how mental and social health and wellbeing are influenced by environmental living conditions. This chapter draws on the current evidence, including WHO task force findings, and examines how the immediate housing environment represents an everyday landscape that can support or limit mental and social wellbeing, in addition to physical health. Addressing housing issues offers public health practitioners an opportunity to target an important social determinant of health. The chapter considers how public health departments can work with local authorities and the voluntary sector to employ multiple strategies to improve housing. These might include developing and enforcing housing guidelines and codes, implementing programmes to improve indoor environmental quality, assessing housing conditions, introducing healthy homes programmes as part of HAZ and advocating healthy, affordable housing. Public health strategies for dealing with homelessness are also discussed.

Key deductions from social context and action in public health

There are a number of conclusions that can be drawn from the theoretical and praxis issues that are given a detailed and critical examination in this book. The first relates to public health policy. There are clearly both challenges and paradoxes presented in some of the policy analysis contained within each of the chapters. What becomes clear is the view that public health in the UK is disadvantaged by its close association with the NHS, with broader public health policy initiatives designed to tackle the wider determinants of health requiring multisector and settings approaches. The evidence of the efficacy of work settings, for example, for the maintenance of health is increasing. It is, of course, rather unfortunate that this is becoming apparent just at the time when the work security of employees is decreasing.

The evidence throughout this text points to a wide range of settings being fundamentally important in addressing the public health needs of the population, not only at a local and national level but also internationally. The dynamics of globalization, for example, and the demographic transition in particular, are forcing changes of priority and practice as population structures and dependency ratios change. To remain proactive in its response to these changes, public health policy must foster strategic alliances on a global scale in which advocacy and effective use of the new electronic media must play an important part. Unfortunately, public health practitioners have been slow to guide mass media presentations towards more structural interpretations of health problems, leaving the field open to programme-makers to use sensationalist and individualist approaches.

Globalization also poses a direct challenge to public health systems that have traditionally concentrated efforts within state borders. There is a need for a paradigm shift to one that focuses action beyond jurisdictional boundaries and nurtures inter agency collaboration.

Another conclusion that can be drawn from the text is that for the social context, social class analysis remains an essential tool if public health practitioners are to understand the dynamics of, and solutions to, tackling health inequalities, both globally and regionally. A key point made is the difficulty in establishing the degree to which inequalities in health between ethnic groups is due to structural differences in power or barriers due to racism.

Alongside ethnicity, public health engagement with disability remains an undeveloped area of practice, perhaps in part because of continuing cultural associations between health, wellbeing and the avoidance of impairment. Part of a solution might reside with disability equality training in which disabled groups engage with the able-bodied, including public health practitioners, to encourage a change of focus from the impaired body to the disabling barriers that generate unnecessary health inequalities.

Strongly aligned to this point, the general welfare and health benefits of social capital and its importance to the reduction of inequalities in health, while often asserted, have remained notoriously difficult to prove. There is a strong confirmation within both parts of this text that social capital does offer health benefits, although differentially distributed by way of status, gender and ethnicity.

Finally, a particularly important conclusion is that the emphasis on the social context of health is moving public health to a more health seeking rather than a disease-avoidance approach. This move towards embracing a more salutogenic philosophy and social model of health to inform action is associated with the new public health movement that arose in the later part of the twentieth century. The challenge will be to sustain these more radical approaches that recognize the wider determinants of health. It is the aim of this text to go some way to encouraging that sustainability.

2 Public health: historical context and current agenda

David Hunter

In the evolution of health policy, concern over the state of the public's health results in public health rising up the policy agenda with governments anxious to demonstrate a commitment not just to making sick people well but to keeping people well and preventing them from falling ill. In many countries, including the UK, we are witnessing one of those periods when public health occupies centre stage (Baggott 2005; Hunter 2005). Such a state of affairs brings with it both opportunities and challenges. Nor is it free from contradictions and paradoxes, as we shall see. Moreover, we have been here before. No sooner has public health achieved prominence than it is just as rapidly relegated to the sidelines, swept aside as the recurring problems of healthcare services reassert themselves and absorb the attention of policy makers.

Not least among the challenges is ensuring that the new-found interest in, and commitment to, public health can be sustained for a sufficient period of time to enable the policy rhetoric to become practical reality. The danger in the fast-moving world of policy change and short-term electoral cycles is that the interest in public health, which demands a long-term commitment, will once again prove short-lived.

This chapter is in two sections. The first reviews the troubled evolution of public health in recent decades in the context of health policies that for the most part have been preoccupied with 'fix and mend' acute healthcare services. This uneasy relationship, or downstream versus upstream tension running through health policy (see Chapter 11 for a further discussion of the terms upstream and downstream), did not always exist, but the uneasy coexistence of public health with healthcare services remains a major concern and arguably constitutes a significant barrier to successful policy implementation (Lewis 1986; Berridge 1999). It constitutes a dominant paradox in view of the unprecedented interest public health has attracted in recent years.

The reasons for this growing interest lie primarily in an acknowledgement of the neglected epidemic of chronic disease, as well as mounting concern over the increasing cost of healthcare services and the need to shift the paradigm towards health improvement and prevention in order to manage demands on healthcare more effectively. Without such a shift, publicly funded health systems are likely to prove unsustainable. At the same time, it has been noted that a widening gap exists between the reality of chronic disease worldwide and the response of national governments to it (Strong *et al.* 2005). Yet, in 2005, all chronic diseases accounted for 72 per cent of the total global burden of disease in the population aged 30 years and older. Chronic disease rates are higher in the Russian Federation and low-income and middle-income countries than in Canada or the UK.

The second section moves from policy to practice and reviews the public health function and whether it is fit for purpose. It takes stock of where we are now and looks ahead to the near future. It explores another tension that has surfaced in public health policy, namely public health as a public good versus the notion that individuals must accept greater responsibility for their health and not rely on government action. Such a distinction goes to the heart of the public health function. In an era of globalization, markets and competition the concept of the public realm urgently needs redefining and possibly rescuing. At a time of growing uncertainty over what we mean by the public good, public health once again finds itself at a crossroads and in danger of losing sight of its purpose and *raison d'être*.

While the focus of the chapter is principally on the UK, where developments have been most marked and well documented and where policy divergence is a feature post-devolution, reference is made where appropriate to developments in Europe and North America, which are struggling with similar concerns and dilemmas.

The evolution of public health policy

The historical review starts in the 1970s. This period witnessed something of an international revival of interest in public health policy and one that echoed what many of the nineteenth century visionaries in public health in the UK already knew, namely the importance of the wider determinants of health and the contribution to health improvement of pure water, effective sewage disposal, food hygiene, decent housing and a safe working environment. In the 1970s, as now, renewed interest in public health was prompted by a number of factors, including the rising costs of healthcare and growing worries about the impact of modern lifestyles on health, the so called diseases of comfort (Baggott 2000; Choi *et al.* 2005).

It proved to be a fertile period in the evolution of public health but also a paradoxical and frustrating one. In terms of policy thinking at this time, the renaissance of public health seemed confident and assured but was in striking contrast to changes occurring in its organization and structure that were having precisely the opposite effect. Public health was at serious risk of losing its way and its ability to implement successfully the policy opportunities that were emerging.

What was to become known as the new public health began in earnest in the 1970s both in the UK and especially in Canada where publication of the Lalonde report heralded a new dawn for public health with its radical and enlightened thinking and critique of modern healthcare systems (Lalonde 1974). The report from the then health minister, Marc Lalonde, proved seminal as it was the first government document to acknowledge that the emphasis in many high-income countries on a biomedical model of healthcare was neither desirable for the enhancement of health nor relevant to prevention. What was radical about the report was its focus on an upstream policy agenda. Future enhancement in the health of Canadians would, it was claimed, come mainly from improvements in the environment, moderating risky lifestyles and increasing our understanding of human biology. Its intellectual underpinnings were inspired by the work of Thomas McKeown, whose thesis was that modern medicine was too disease-focused and overly concerned with the individual at the expense of taking a holistic view (McKeown 1979). It ignored the wider socioeconomic and environmental determinants of health.

The Lalonde report introduced the health field concept as the basis for rebalancing health policy away from a preoccupation with healthcare and towards a concern with the environment and lifestyle. The health field concept was not faultless and attracted its critics who took issue with the, in their view, misplaced emphasis on lifestyle factors which could lead to victim blaming (Ryan 1976) by attempting to persuade individuals to take responsibility for their own health while ignoring that they are victims of structural circumstances. Socioeconomic and environmental factors as key determinants of health received insufficient attention. Not all the factors and pressures affecting health status were amenable to individual influence or decision. Over 30 years later, similar heated debates between the collective and individual continue to rage and shape policy, as we shall see below.

Whatever its shortcomings, the Lalonde report became a touchstone for all those reformers committed to a whole systems approach to health policy in which there was a search for a new equilibrium between healthcare considerations and those affecting the wider health of the population. Sadly, since the Lalonde report, progress has been un-derwhelming and, as Legowski and McKay (2000) have concluded, there has been a logjam in health policy. In the end, Lalonde failed to break the mould or shift the policy paradigm, and the prevailing bias in favour of healthcare services and the vested interests associated with them has continued more or less unabated.

Elsewhere, like the UK, the policy response to the new public health thinking was far less ambitious. Like Lalonde, the equivalent report from the government, published in 1976, was a product of economic restraint and pressures on resources (DHSS 1976). Unlike Lalonde, its impact remained muted. It did not make specific recommendations for policy change but was intended merely to start people thinking and talking about the place of prevention in the overall, longer-term development of the health and related services. Nevertheless, it sought to stress the message that prevention is better than cure and paved the way some 16 years later for the first ever health strategy for England.

The Health of the Nation

The first health strategy in England, *The Health of the Nation* (*HOTN*), appeared in 1992 (DoH 1992). It was preceded some years earlier by the first health strategy in the UK produced by the devolved administration responsible for health in Wales (Welsh Health Planning Forum 1989a, 1989b). The *HOTN* was remarkable not only for being the first strategy of its kind but for being produced by a Conservative government not renowned for its commitment either to central planning or to the broader health agenda. This was, after all, a government that did not subscribe to the notion of health inequalities or believe that poverty might have something to do with the widening health gap between social groups. Up until then, most of the government's energies had been devoted to introducing an internal market into the National Health Service (NHS). The attempt to talk publicly about the importance of health rather than healthcare echoed the discussions in the 1970s at the time of the Lalonde report. Upon its publication, health ministers and officials insisted that *HOTN* was 'shifting the focus from NHS institutions and service inputs to people and health' (Mawhinney and Nichol 1993: 45). The *HOTN* also sought to widen the responsibility for health across government, although its origins were firmly rooted in the Department of Health (DoH) and the NHS, who were regarded as the natural leaders in public health.

There was also an international significance to the *HOTN*. It acknowledged its debt to the World Health Organization's (WHO) *Health for All* approach (WHO 1985) in its overarching goal to add years to life and life to years. In turn, the WHO cited the *HOTN* as a model strategy which demonstrated how governments could act to improve population health.

The *HOTN* was generally welcomed although not devoid of criticism, which centred on two issues: its failure to take into account socioeconomic determinants of health, and the pursuit of a largely disease based model of health in respect of the strategy's thrust and the targets set. Some argued that the targets and activities should focus on the factors that led to ill health, such as smoking, poverty, inadequate housing, for example, rather than on the diseases and conditions that resulted (Holland and Stewart 1998).

The *HOTN* heralded a commitment to target setting that was to remain a feature of all subsequent health strategies, and, indeed, of public policy more generally under subsequent governments. Such an overly prescriptive approach to managing performance, whereby targets were determined by the centre and imposed on health authorities, was criticized for being inflexible and inhibiting implementation (Barnes and Rathwell 1993; Hunter 2002). Such an approach was also felt to concentrate on the measurable to the exclusion of the unmeasurable.

Despite its significance as, in the words of the National Audit Office, an ambitious and far-reaching strategy, the implementation of the *HOTN* proved less successful (DoH 1998). When the performance of the NHS was being judged, the *HOTN* did not seem to figure. What mattered far more were the by now familiar preoccupations with reducing waiting lists, ensuring speedy access to hospital beds and keeping within budget. Whenever the going got tough, public health would be among the first casualties as managers focused on the priorities affecting acute care services. They were not held to account for failing to meet *HOTN* targets. Little has changed over the years in this respect (Hunter and Marks 2005).

New government, new strategies

New Labour entered office in May 1997 promising a paradigm shift in health policy. Not only would there be no more radical structural reforms of the NHS, but also at the top of its priorities would be public health. To emphasize the point, a new post of public health minister was created in England but not elsewhere in the UK. Political devolution to Wales, Scotland and Northern Ireland in 2000 meant that health policy became a devolved responsibility with political leadership being exercised from Cardiff, Edinburgh and Belfast.

The new Labour government on taking office in the late 1990s was keen to show its commitment to a more socially equitable and cohesive society that involved the efforts of all government departments and not only health. It became publicly acceptable to talk about health inequalities and the social determinants of health. A range of policies, including Sure Start (see Chapter 13), the welfare to work programme, tax credits, national minimum wage and national strategy for neighbourhood renewal (see Chapter 14), were all intended to tackle social deprivation and poor health.

As part of its determination to do things differently, the public health minister commissioned a review of the evidence base in tackling health inequalities in order to advise where government should focus its attention (DoH 1998). Of the review's 39 recommendations, only three directly concerned the NHS or were within its power to influence directly (Macintyre 2000).

Part of the government's response lay in producing a successor strategy to the *HOTN* (DoH 1999). Although the strategy was concerned with settings in health, like the workplace (see Chapter 15), school and community, some commentators were disappointed that it belonged firmly to a healthcare model which was less about supporting communities to remain healthy than about keeping individuals alive (Fulop and Hunter 1999). Repeating a perceived flaw in the *HOTN*, the new strategy was focused mainly on disease based areas such as cancer, coronary heart disease/stroke, and mental illness, with targets similarly disease based. Just as the *HOTN* found that the dominance of the medical model underlying it proved to be a major barrier to its ownership by agencies outside the health sector, notably local government and voluntary agencies, so a similar fate seemed destined to befall its successor.

The appearance of a new strategy to replace the *HOTN* did not complete the government's public health policy making, far from it. As the government moved into a new decade and century, the flow of policies increased with an urgency and energy that rather bewildered managers and practitioners among others. A key development in thinking about public health was the work of Derek Wanless, former chair of the National Westminster Bank, who was invited by the Chancellor of the Exchequer to advise on future health trends over a 20-year period and on the ability of a health service funded by central taxation to meet whatever challenges lay ahead.

In the first of two reports, Wanless gave an unexpected prominence to the importance of public health. His argument was that health and wealth went together: good health relies on good economics. More specifically, the report maintained that 'better public health measures could significantly affect the demand for health care' (Wanless 2002: 1.27). On top of any health benefits, a focus on public health was seen to bring wider benefits by increasing productivity and reducing inactivity in the working age population. In terms of the overall balance of care, Wanless was critical of the prevailing bias in favour of acute hospital care.

Such a bias in health policy is by no means peculiar to the UK. The WHO in its *World Health Report 2002* points out that much scientific effort and most health resources are directed towards treating disease rather than preventing it (WHO 2002). It calls on governments, in their stewardship role, to achieve a much better balance between preventing disease and merely treating its consequences. Lack of political will, not knowledge, is hindering progress.

The government accepted the Wanless analysis and recommendation that the government act to reduce demand on healthcare by promoting health. However, the programme was an ambitious one and required a step change in the delivery of health policy.

Indeed, so keen was the government to demonstrate its commitment to a new approach and to a rebalancing of health policy in the direction charted by Wanless that he was invited to review progress the following year. It was of course far too soon to make robust judgements about the success of his strategy, but in his second report, Wanless (2004) focused on the public health system in its widest sense and produced a powerful critique of the public health function, a point picked up later in this chapter.

The government's response to Wanless's second report was to deflect attention from it by immediately announcing that a new health strategy would be produced to which the public would be invited to contribute through a major consultation exercise. Many public health practitioners and policy commentators queried whether a new strategy was required since the existing one, *Saving Lives: Our Healthier Nation*, had yet to be implemented and had already suffered from being sidelined by the priority targets in healthcare services, none of which affected public health.

In late 2004 the government published its new health strategy for England, *Choosing Health: Making Healthy Choices Easier* (DoH 2004). It marked a significant departure in terms of how the government saw its role in health improvement. Whereas its earlier strategy had emphasized the dual approach between government and individuals in promoting health, the new strategy shifted the focus much more firmly and explicitly towards the individual. The language around choice and for individual responsibility in leading healthier lives was new and, rather than government exercising a leadership role, as envisaged in *Our Healthier Nation* and in the WHO's health development report, the role of government had been recast as a more modest enabling, facilitating one designed to provide advice and information in order to support individuals in making healthier choices. It marked a significant shift in public health thinking, albeit one in keeping with the government's approach in general to public policy and public-sector reform. What has been termed the marketization of policy was being applied to health as it was to other areas of government policy including the NHS itself (Hunter 2005). From about 2002, the government's reform rhetoric centred on devolution, putting power back to the front line, reducing central control, and giving patients and public more choice. The 1999 health strategy clearly needed updating to reflect the new language of political discourse and to bring thinking into line with the new mantra of choice and market style incentives to modify lifestyles. Such thinking also dominates the most recent health policy strategy which is concerned with shifting the balance from hospital to primary and community care (Secretary of State for Health 2005). As the strategy acknowledges, the issues raised are pertinent to public health since they are aimed at keeping people healthy and out of institutional care.

The example of the ban on smoking in public places illustrates the difference in approach well and the cautious nature of public health policy. In keeping with its emphasis on individual choice and desire not to be accused of being the nanny state, the English government was reluctant to take a lead on banning smoking. It was only when pressure began to mount, aided by a decision to ban smoking in Northern Ireland, Scotland and Wales, that ministers felt compelled to follow suit in England. However, even then the government left it to an open vote in Parliament to decide (see Chapter 17 for a full discussion of the government's efforts on smoking).

Developments in Wales and Scotland

The arrival of political devolution in 2000 gave a new impetus to UK health policy. At the time of writing, Northern Ireland remains something of a special case, pending a resolution of the political difficulties there. Until such time the devolved assembly has been suspended.

To a greater degree than is evident in England, Wales and Scotland have sought in their respective strategies to put health before healthcare (see for example National Assembly for Wales 2001; Scottish Executive 2003). What remains unclear is whether the strong rhetoric is, or will be, matched by developments on the ground. Greer (2001), who has studied the development of public health in the devolved polities, is sceptical, claiming that Scotland is speaking of public health but still focusing on healthcare services, and Wales is focusing on integrated public health activities and promotion. It is also the case that Wales suffers from severe financial problems in its healthcare services that may prove too distracting to ignore in favour of putting health first.

It remains early days as far as devolution is concerned and as to whether it will result in a marked divergence in health policy as distinct from what happened under the former system of administrative devolution when policies and reforms varied at the margin but rarely in substance or in principle (Hunter and Wistow 1987; Hazell and Jervis 1998). Certainly, in respect of the smoking ban Scotland has shown the way within the UK (see Chapter 17) and it seems likely that this may encourage the Scottish Executive to show similar bold leadership in respect of, for example, obesity. There is certainly talk of linking public health challenges to agendas around social justice and environmental sustainability. Despite much discussion of the need to merge these agendas, progress has been slow in England. It would be far easier to make the connections in the smaller UK countries. Moreover, while issues of globalization are as evident in Scotland and Wales as they are in England, the language of choice, markets and competition is absent from public discourse. There appears still to be a belief in, and support for, a public realm and a role for government in promoting the public good that remains distinctive. In these ways, at least, significant differences are evident across the UK.

Developments outside the UK

These issues are by no means confined to the UK. In the USA, for example, a report from the Institute of Medicine (IOM) on the future of the public's health concluded that the USA is not fully meeting its potential in the area of population health (IOM 2003). It argued that the public's health could be supported only through collective action, not through individual endeavour. The collective goods that are essential conditions for health can be secured only through organized action on behalf of the population (Gostin 2000). The IOM report asserted that health is a primary public good because many aspects of human potential such as employment, social relationships and political participation are contingent on it. Creating the conditions for people to be healthy should therefore be a shared social goal and government had a special role in this together with the contributions of other sectors of society.

A review of policies across Europe to tackle health inequalities found that despite some progress, many challenges remained (Judge *et al.* 2005). In particular, policies needed to be supported by financial and political commitment as well as steps being taken to ensure that adequate capacity and infrastructure were in place to allow effective implementation to occur. It is to such matters we now turn.

Regardless of the precise nature of a policy or strategy, and the support that exists for it, if the means to implement it are either non existent or inadequate in terms of capacity or capability or both then it will count for little. Wanless (2004) was struck by the mismatch between policy statements accumulating over some 30 years and a persistent failure to secure their rigorous implementation. The next section considers the public health function and its fitness for purpose.

The public health function

Traditionally, public health has maintained close links with medicine although notions like the new public health or wider public health have been employed to demonstrate that the actions of many other professions and organizations have as much influence, and possibly more, on health improvement than an exclusively medical model of public health. The proximity of public health to medicine and healthcare remains an un-comfortable one in respect of public health interventions aimed at tackling the social determinants of health. The proximity has also resulted in public health being repeatedly overshadowed by more urgent issues arising from the acute healthcare sector. In Wan-less's words, 'in spite of numerous policy initiatives being directed towards public health, they have not resulted in a rebalancing of policy away from health care' (Wanless 2004: 38).

In the UK until 1974, public health practitioners were located in local government, a location that many regarded as more appropriate for the pursuit of the health of a popu-lation than a place in the NHS which was dominated by the service needs of individual patients. But the first major reorganization of the NHS in 1974 saw public health, or community medicine as it was then called, move from local government to the NHS where the key tensions between healthcare and health came to the surface. They were inevitable under an arrangement whereby the management and leadership of public health resided with the healthcare system whose leaders had little understanding or knowledge of public health. The hope was that the new specialty would take its rightful place alongside general practice and hospital medicine and compete for resources on equal terms. But things turned out rather differently and the legacy of that reorganization remains alive in current debates about the public health function.

These debates were revisited in the House of Commons Health Committee's 2000–1 inquiry into public health (House of Commons Health Committee 2001). While a few of the Committee's members, including its then chair, were sympathetic to the notion of returning public health to local government, it was persuaded by the weight of written and oral evidence that the issues were not primarily ones of organizational structure or where functions were located but had much more to do with effective leadership, poli-tical will and a genuine commitment to partnership working. Gaining wider acceptance for public health as a core part of local government is seen as the key to wresting re-sponsibility away from the NHS where public health has a habit of being subsumed within a model that focuses on sickness and ill health (Elson 2004).

Nevertheless, there remain tensions and an underlying sense that as long as the lead responsibility for public health remains with the NHS then, in the words of the Health Committee, 'it runs the risk of trailing well behind fix and mend medical services' (House of Commons Health Committee 2001: para. 47). Many commentators, including Wanless, have also argued that while a major contributor, the NHS is only one element of the public health delivery system. An essential element, in Wanless's view, is the recognition that the greatest contribution to public health is made by individuals in the wider public health workforce, many of whom have job titles that do not mention public health, or even health (Wanless 2004).

Epping-Jordan *et al.* (2005) support this view and argue that intersectoral action is necessary at all stages of policy formulation and implementation in respect of chronic disease, as the major determinants lie outside the health sector (for further discussion on intersectoral action and policy, see Chapter 11).

That there were deficits in the structure and functioning of public health in the UK was reaffirmed in the Chief Medical Officer's (CMO) public health function review published at the same time as the Health Committee's report (DoH 2001). The function review was undertaken in response to the government's desire to improve the health of the population as a whole but especially that of the worst-off sections of society. Implementation, it was argued, would not succeed without a strong public health function equipped with the requisite skills and competencies. Doubts had been expressed over whether the function was fit for purpose. Five major themes emerged as essential for a successful public health function:

- a wider understanding of health and wellbeing;
- better coordination and communication within the public health function;
- effective joined up working;
- sustained community development and public involvement;
- an increase in capacity and capabilities in the public health function.

The CMO's report was accompanied by suspicions that it was merely an exercise in going through the motions rather than heralding the start of a significant new phase in the evolution of public health. In particular, was it simply another example of symbolic policy making and gesture politics from which public health seemed to suffer more than its fair share?

Evidence to support this assessment of the function review came a few years later in the Wanless report on public health. In a wide-ranging critique of the failure of public health to deliver despite numerous policy statements, Wanless (2004: 70) concluded that 'developments to strengthen public health capacity need to address both the knowledge and competence of individual members of the workforce, and the capacity of organisations to support and deliver public health activity'.

In addition, the IOM report found that a number of systemic problems were evident in explaining the shortcomings of America's public health system. Problems of underfunding, fragmentation and lack of coordination at all levels of government had 'dire consequences for the public's health' (IOM 2003: 26). The report adopted the concept of a public health system to describe a complex network of individuals and organizations that have the potential to play critical roles in creating conditions for health.

As the previous section showed, we have reached a stage in England where the whole concept of the public realm is being challenged if not undermined by business notions of what constitutes successful governance. The blurring of the public private boundary in areas like health in the interests of abandoning ideology and supporting what works may, however unwittingly, be making the job of public health and its practitioners increasingly problematic.

Writing about the crisis of public health, Julio Frenk, a public health academic who is now Mexico's health minister, noted that public health has historically been one of the vital forces leading to collective action for health and wellbeing. However, the widespread impression exists today that this leading role has been weakening and that public health is experiencing a severe identity crisis and a crisis of organization and accomplishment (Frenk 1992).

Such a crisis is evident in many countries and stems broadly from the same causes alluded to above. The paradox is that at precisely the time when the challenges facing the public's health, whether obesity, alcohol consumption, sexual health or narrowing the health gap between social groups, demand healthy public policy (see Chapter 11), governments seem to be retreating from their responsibilities and claiming that it is all too difficult and that change can be forthcoming only through individuals acting as consumers and expressing their desires in the marketplace. Where this leaves public health poses a dilemma, especially when much public health practice in the UK is already systemically weakened by being bound up with the fate of the NHS (Berridge 1999; Hunter 2003). One way forward would be for the public health community to exercise more political leverage and advocate for what it believes in, including encouraging local government to assume a stronger leadership role as favoured by Elson (2004).

But the challenge goes further and is succinctly expressed by the Institute of Medicine (IOM) in its report on the future of the public's health, when arguing that meaningful protection and assurance of the population's health requires communal effort from multiple actors and organizations (IOM 2003).

There are limits to markets and to viewing individuals as consumers exercising unfettered choice. Other conceptions of modernity exist. It is perhaps time for public health to acknowledge this and to exercise whatever influences it can muster.

References

Baggott, R. (2000) *Public Health: Policy and Politics*. London: Palgrave Macmillan.

Baggott, R. (2005) From sickness to health? Public health in England, *Public Money & Management*, 25: 229–36.

Barnes, R. and Rathwell, T. (1993) *Study to Assess Progress in the Adoption and Implementation of Health Goals and Targets at the Regional and Local Levels*. Leeds: Nuffield Institute for Health, University of Leeds.

Berridge, V. (1999) *Health and Society in Britain since 1939*. Cambridge: Cambridge University Press.

Choi, B.C.K., Hunter, D.J., Tsou, W. and Sainsbury, P. (2005) Diseases of comfort: primary cause of death in the 22nd century, *Journal of Epidemiology & Community Health*, 59: 1030–4.

DHSS (Department of Health and Social Security) (1976) *Prevention and Health: Everybody's Business: A Reassessment of Public and Personal Health*. London: HMSO.

DoH (Department of Health) (1992) *The Health of the Nation: A Strategy for Health in England*, Cm 1986. London: HMSO.

DoH (Department of Health) (1998) *The Health of the Nation – A Policy Assessed*. London: HMSO.

DoH (Department of Health) (1999) *Saving Lives: Our Healthier Nation*, Cm 4386. London: HMSO.

DoH (Department of Health) (2001) *The Report of the Chief Medical Officer's Project to Strengthen the Public Health Function*. London: HMSO.

DoH (Department of Health) (2004) *Choosing Health: Making Healthy Choices Easier*. London: HMSO.

Elson, T. (2004) Why public health must become a core part of council agendas, in K. Skinner (ed.) *Community Leadership and Public Health: The Role of Local Authorities*. London: The Smith Institute.

Epping-Jordan, J., Galia, G., Tukuitonga, C. and Beaglehole, R. (2005) Preventing chronic diseases: taking stepwise action, *The Lancet*, 5 October (published online).

Frenk, J. (1992) The new public health, in Pan American Health Organization (ed.) *The Crisis of Public Health: Reflections for the Debate*. Washington: PAHO.

Fulop, N. and Hunter, D.J. (1999) Editorial: saving lives or sustaining the public's health? *British Medical Journal*, 319: 139–40.

Gostin, L.O. (2000) *Public Health Law: Power, Duty, Restraint*. Berkeley, CA: University of California Press and Milbank Memorial Fund.

Greer, S. (2001) *Divergence and Devolution*. London: The Nuffield Trust.

Hazell, R. and Jervis, P. (1998) *Devolution and Health*. London: The Nuffield Trust.

Holland, W.W. and Stewart, S. (1998) *Public Health: The Vision and the Challenge*. London: The Nuffield Trust.

House of Commons Health Committee (2001) *Public Health*. Second Report. Volume I: Report and Proceedings of the Committee. Session 2000–01, HC30-II. London: HMSO.

Hunter, D.J. (2002) England, in M. Marinker (ed.) *Health Targets in Europe: Polity, Progress and Promise*. London: BMJ Books.

Hunter, D.J. (2003) *Public Health Policy*. Cambridge: Polity.

Hunter, D.J. (2005) Choosing or losing health? *Journal of Epidemiology & Community Health*, 59: 1010–12.

Hunter, D.J. and Marks, L. (2005) *Managing for Health: What Incentives Exist for NHS Managers to Focus on Wider Health Issues?* London: King's Fund.

Hunter, D.J. and Wistow, G. (1987) The paradox of policy diversity in a unitary state: community care in Britain, *Public Administration*, 65: 3–24.

IOM (Institute of Medicine) (2003) *The Future of the Public's Health in the 21st Century*. Washington: National Academy Press.

Judge, K., Platt, S., Costongs, C. and Jurczak, K. (2005) *Health Inequalities: A Challenge for Europe*. London: UK Presidency of the EU.

Lalonde, M. (1974) *A New Perspective on the Health of Canadians*. Ottawa: Minister of Supply and Services.

Legowski, B. and McKay, L. (2000) *Health Beyond Health Care: Twenty-Five Years of Federal Health Policy Development*. CPRN Discussion Paper No. H/04. Ottawa: Canadian Policy Research Networks.

Lewis, J. (1986) *What Price Community Medicine? The Philosophy, Practice and Politics of Public Health Since 1919*. Brighton: Wheatsheaf.

Macintyre, S. (2000) Modernising the NHS: prevention and the reduction of health inequalities, *British Medical Journal*, 320: 1399–400.

McKeown, T. (1979) *The Role of Medicine: Dream, Mirage or Nemesis,* 2nd edn. Oxford: Blackwell.

Mawhinney, B. and Nichol, D. (1993) *Purchasing for Health: A Framework for Action.* London: NHS Management Executive.

National Assembly for Wales (2001) *Improving Health in Wales: A Plan for the NHS with its Partners.* Cardiff: National Assembly for Wales.

Ryan, W. (1976) *Blaming the Victim.* New York: Vintage Books.

Scottish Executive (2003) *Improving Health in Scotland – the Challenge.* Edinburgh: Scottish Executive.

Secretary of State for Health (2005) *Our Health, Our Care, Our Say: A New Direction for Community Services,* Cm 6737. London: HMSO.

Strong, K., Mathers, C., Leeder, S. and Beaglehole, R. (2005) Preventing chronic diseases: how many lives can we save? *The Lancet,* 5 October (published online).

Wanless, D. (2002) *Securing our Future Health: Taking a Long-Term View.* Final report. London: HM Treasury.

Wanless, D. (2004) *Securing Good Health for the Whole Population.* Final report. London: HM Treasury and Department of Health.

Welsh Health Planning Forum (1989a) *Strategic Intent and Direction for the NHS in Wales.* Cardiff: Welsh Office.

Welsh Health Planning Forum (1989b) *Local Strategies for Health: A New Approach to Strategic Planning.* Cardiff: Welsh Office.

WHO (World Health Organization) (1985) *Targets for Health for All.* Copenhagen: WHO Regional Office for Europe.

WHO (World Health Organization) (2002) *The World Health Report 2002: Reducing Risks, Promoting Healthy Life.* Geneva: WHO.

Part 1
The social context of public health

3 Trends and transitions: the sociopolitical context of public health

Sebastian Garman

Whether regarded as a theory, model or set of interlinked generalizations (Kirk 1996) the demographic transition remains an influential starting point for a discussion of the sociopolitical context of public health. With early versions deriving from the 1940s it has continued to order debate and help anticipate social trends and problems that impact upon public health decision making (for a comprehensive critical overview see Chesnais 1992) for half a century. Demographic transition theory comprises many versions but what all have in common is the attempt to generalize about the process by which premodern mainly agrarian societies, typified by relatively high fertility and high death rates, seem to move through a series of stages to a postulated stability of postmodern urban industrial societies typified by low birth rates and low death rates. It is the changing political dynamics caused by the shifting sizes of cohorts, whether of age, gender, class or ethnicity as well as the concomitant changes in social institution that is of significance to public health.

The age cohorts of the demographic transition can be represented graphically as a move from the shape of a stepped pyramid, with a broad base of younger population cohorts surmounted by ever smaller cohorts of older people, via an onion shape caused by the shrinkage of the base as each generation has fewer children, to the final shape of a column, where each age cohort is of a similar size.

Figure 3.1, for example, juxtaposes the pyramid shape for Great Britain for the year 1821 against a transition shape halfway between an onion and a column for the year 2004. One thing immediately becomes clear from these graphics: the demographic transition implies a radical restructuring of intergenerational politics and identity with the consequent ageing structure of populations. Within the UK, for example, where there were 14.3 million young people under 16 in 1971, there were 11.6 million in 2004 and are projected to be 11.2 million by the year 2011, a decline of some 20 per cent. In the same period those aged 65 and over have increased in number from 7.4 million in 1971 to 9.6 million in 2004 and are projected to increase further to 10.5 million by 2011 and 12.7 million by the year 2021, an increase of some 50 per cent (ONS 2006). These ageing population structures are replicated across Europe with Italy, Germany and Greece having the highest proportion of older people and Ireland the lowest. The pattern is being extended rapidly to the rest of the world.

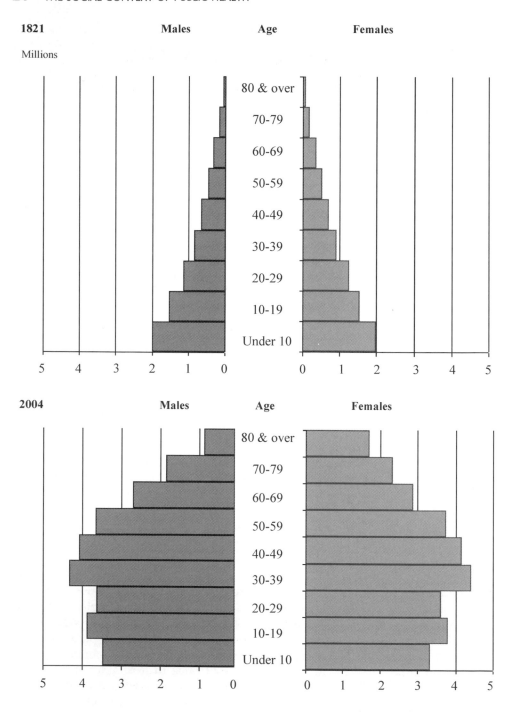

Figure 3.1 Population by sex and age for Great Britain, 1821 and 2004
Source: ONS (2006); General Register Office for Scotland

The demographic transition in its seminal formulations has been regarded as having four stages: a preliminary fall in mortality rates, a consequential rise in population, a later fall in fertility rates with a final balancing or even a decrease of population size. There has been much debate about the causal factors at work here.

Mortality and fertility

For the initial strategic fall in mortality, particularly infant and maternal mortality, improvements of diet, hygiene, water supply and sanitation were important causal factors as well as the growth of public order, communications and social administration (Schofield *et al.* 1991; Kirk 1996). These gains in lives saved were consolidated through the latter part of the nineteenth century and much of the twentieth century by an era of rapid advances in knowledge and technique of biomedicine. This continual reduction in death rates, in the UK for all ages except early adulthood, has helped maintain population growth in mature nation states with industrial economies and has thus delayed the completion of the demographic transition to a period of predicted population decline. By the latter part of the twentieth century this effect, however, was largely over in the UK and northwest Europe where further decreases in mortality now make populations older (Coleman 2000).

The aetiology of the fall in fertility is particularly interesting for what it implies about gender, power and politics. Demographic transitions are occurring globally with an initial decline in mortality followed by rapid population growth and a later decline in fertility. Yet here the period of the transition is much quicker than it was for western Europe and is occurring in societies with very different levels of economic and social development by a process that must include an important element of innovation and diffusion (see Kirk 1996 for an influential overview). Nevertheless a strategic causal factor of self interest seems to be important everywhere. In traditional agrarian societies women tended to live shorter lives than men, but wherever industrialism and the process of modernity have occurred women now live longer than men (Shorter 1983). In agrarian societies the incentive to restrict family size, where it exists at all, is very indirect; guided by social mores, such as those governing sexual relations, and institutions like the delaying of marriage or monasticism. Moreover women have little personal control over their fertility. Quite apart from the improved technologies of contraception by which women gain some control over their bodies, industrialism, labour markets and the individualist rewards of consumerism can cause the incentive to restrict family size to become very personal and direct. Strategic to these changes in Europe was the increasing relative cost of children and their removal from the process of maintaining economic support for parents (Gillis *et al.* 1992) by way of institutions such as compulsory full time education.

Within Britain the key years of fertility decline were between the 1870s and the 1920s, from an average of six children ever born to around two, as contraception became accepted and available. The lowest point of this trend was in 1933 with a recorded total fertility ratio (TFR) of 1.72 (Coleman 2000). Between the 1930s and the 1970s there followed a period of volatility through much of Europe with baby booms and busts as parents took advantage of their unprecedented powers to control the pace and outcome of childbearing. Since that time fertility rates in northwest Europe have been fairly steady (1.7–2.0 TFR), if below replacement levels. Elsewhere in Europe the instability persists, with quite dramatic falls in fertility in eastern Europe with the collapse of communism, while in southern Europe Italy and Spain have recorded some of the lowest birth rates in the world (1.2–1.3 TFR).

Apart from its aberrant US like pattern of teenage births, the British trends in fertility are fairly typical of the rest of northwest Europe with large numbers of women delaying births until their late thirties or remaining childless. The social institution of marriage as a constraint on fertility gave way in the second part of the twentieth century until, by 1999, in the UK a third of births occurred outside marriage and cohabitation had become the normal practice before marriage. Here the UK pattern is fairly typical of both Europe and America, being midway between the Nordic countries, where well over 40 per cent of births in 1999 were outside marriage and the southern European pattern of Italy and Greece, along with Switzerland, where 10 per cent or less of births occurred outside marriage (Kiernan 2004). Of interest to demographers for more than a century because of its significance for fertility, marriage has become increasingly irrelevant in this respect in both northern Europe and America. Social scientists have turned their attention to the psychological and social costs of marriage breakdown to both adults and children. For example, in a study of ten European nations as well as the USA the findings are robust and clear. Using 1990s data it was found that in every nation studied children of divorced parents were more likely to form partnerships and to bear children at a young age; were more likely to cohabit rather than marry; were less likely to have their first child in marriage; and to form partnerships themselves that were more likely to break up (Kiernan 2004; for a discussion of the success of public health policy in the UK in attempts to support families and children see Chapter 13).

Yet as the author herself concludes, the anxieties caused by such comparisons (for example see Waite and Gallagher 2000) might well be misplaced since cohabitation is only recently emerging as a social institution subject to communal mores and public expectations. Indeed, a simple comparison between cohabiting unions and marriages is not comparing like with like since more stable cohabiting unions are often converted into marriage. It is perhaps more interesting to compare national cultures where cohabitation appears to be becoming a successful institutional alternative to marriage, particularly where children are involved, as in some Nordic countries and in France. It then becomes apparent that in Britain and the USA, families with dependent children, whether based on marriage or on cohabitation, have higher dissolution rates and there are more solo mothers and teenage pregnancies in these countries (Kiernan 2004).

Migration

Early versions of the demographic transition theory failed to take account of the importance to communication of aspects of globalization, such as trade and the impact of the digital revolution on the mediation and diffusion of ideas (for further examination of the impact of globalization on public health see Chapter 10). More specifically it has become increasingly apparent that migration effects the process in two ways. On the one hand, disparities in global economic and population growth rates combined with rapidly increasing global communications are increasing the pressures of migration from low income high birth rate regions to high income low birth rate regions with relative labour shortages (McCarthy 2001; GCIM 2005). On the other hand, the impact of migration on high income countries is slowing the process of ageing population structures and the predicted population decline.

Within the UK, for example, the delay in the completion of the demographic transition has not only been due to the lowering of mortality rates in the twentieth century and the particularly large postwar baby boom which ended in 1965, it has also been substantially influenced by migration. Through much of the nineteenth century the UK was a net exporter of people to countries with which it had colonial or imperial ties. This substantially lowered the effects of the rapid population growth, with for example a net benefit to North America of some 3 million, mainly young, people in the nineteenth century (Coleman 2000).

Since the 1960s, however, the flow of migrants has been substantially inwards with marked effects on population size and growth so that now migration accounts for about half of UK population increase (ONS 2006). Half of all gross migration flows into the UK since the 1960s have been from the new Commonwealth and there has also been a 30 year rising trend in migration from continental Europe, made easier by the Single European Act of 1985. According to official figures, adjusting for visitor switchers, net immigration increased unevenly, but by the late 1990s it was over 100,000 per year. In the latest estimates of 2004 the figure had risen to 222,600 per annum, 71,600 people more than in 2003 (ONS 2006). Moreover there are considerable doubts about the reliability of official figures highlighted by, for example, the discrepancies in records about failed asylum seekers where it was recently suggested by the Home Office that there are 400,000 to 450,000 case files on failed applications, far more than the 283,500 estimated by the National Audit Office in 2005 (NAO 2005; Reuters 2006). Between 2004 and 2006 the number of migrant workers from the eight new accession countries of the European Union (EU) was estimated to be some 600,000. Immigrant populations tend to be young in age with higher fertility rates and so they have an increasingly significant impact on total population fertility as well as, of course, increasing the total. The dramatic variations in estimates of immigration over the last four years in the UK is leading to difficulties in projections and planning (for the basis of orthodox government projections, see GAD 2005; for a critique of GAD estimates see Migration Watch 2006) for health, welfare, housing and education requirements (for a different focus on population mobility and public health see Chapter 7).

Public health implications

For high income nation states, particularly those towards the end of the demographic transition such as those of northwest Europe, Canada and Japan, mortality rates have dropped to such a low level that any further gains will be marginal in their effect on population structures. Fertility rates are below the rate of replacement, inward migration is on a rising trend and populations are rapidly ageing.

In the most general policy terms there is widespread recognition that the future of public health policy depends on moving resources from individualized hospital-based medicine into less expensive community-based health promotion strategies focused on self support and self reliance (see for example DoH 2004). More specifically there is a far greater understanding of the economics of the elderly dependency ratio (Stolnitz 1994), particularly with the relatively new methodology of generational accounting. The elderly dependency ratio, defined as those over 60 years old as a share of the working-age population (20–59), is estimated to increase from 37 per cent in 1995 to 47 per cent in 2015 and to 67 per cent in 2035 on an EU average. Generational accounting is a way of calculating the costs to each living generation of the payment of governmental bills incurred by governments on their behalf. The room for manoeuvre of governments in planning taxation depends in large part on the interaction between the dynamics of the demographic transition and their indebtedness (see Kotlikoff and Raffelhuschen 1999). Thus a more strategic ratio is that of the number of persons contributing to the pension schemes to those drawing on them. This is expected to fall in the UK below 2:1 by the year 2020 (Coleman 2000) unless counteracted by a fairly continuous inward migration of youthful labour.

The first great fall in fertility rates in the UK, between the 1870s and the 1930s, with its low point of 1933, occurred during the first experiment in economic globalization with open markets and peaks of migration (James 2001). This experiment collapsed in the Great Depression among boundary fears of otherness and aliens: the suicide of the race, miscegenation, laws against migrants, and calls for the promotion of eugenics (Hunt 1999). The present fall in European fertility has led to no such political ramifications although there are heightened fears of boundaries and ethnicity which, if accompanied by an economic recession and large rises in unemployment, could be serious.

Other anxieties have focused on identity and social order, particularly in the context of changes to family and marriage, civic identity, social coherence and communal ties. In the early twentieth century such concerns tended to focus around the unfortunately named moral, social or racial hygiene movements (Hunt 1999). It is interesting that the dialogue now tends to be framed at the level of individual and family responsibility without a counterbalancing consideration of the changing social structures such as the effect of neo liberal economics on civic institutions supporting social cohesion (for further consideration of these ideas see Chapters 5 and 6).

The epidemiological transition

The demographic transition radically alters the patterns of disease and death, forcing large adjustments in policy towards public health. The notion of the epidemiological transition has arisen to describe this process as epidemiologists attempt to model and test the observation that as mortality rates fall and populations age the cause of death shifts from communicable to noncommunicable diseases (Salomon and Murray 2002) or, as some variants suggest, a more intricate interaction between falls in fertility rates and falls in mortality rates and changing disease patterns, particularly those of children (see Albala and Vio 1995). Deriving from a seminal paper (see Omran 2005) interest has focused as much on the cultural dynamics and changes of value orientations of populations as on an attempt to describe the changing patterns of mortality. Indeed, some researchers use the more embracing notion of the health transition (Caldwell 1993) to include consideration of the interactions of the changing patterns of disease and changes in health service provision.

Before examining the implications of these changes it would be wise to register a caveat: just as the adoption of contemporary ways of life should not be held responsible for increased mortality from degenerative diseases, so a concern about lifestyle diseases should not be at the cost of vigilance in the face of recurrent communicable diseases. The demographic transition model records changes in proportion: degenerative diseases have always been significant, but they were less evident to earlier generations because of the much higher incidence of communicable diseases at that time (Gage 1993; Kirk 1996), and communicable diseases are a very real threat now, so much so that some have coined the expression, 'the third epidemiological transition', to describe the risk (see for example Barrett *et al.* 1998; for further discussion see Chapter 10). Within Europe, heightened risks of communicable disease have been managed in part by a network approach, although funding difficulties might endanger the exercise (MacLehose *et al.* 2002; McKee 2005) and the collapse of the former Soviet Union has led to special challenges in international cooperation. A good recent case is the danger of avian influenza. Certain countries have broadcast management strategies such as that of Canada (Health Canada 2004). It has been suggested, however, that most have neither planned for the dangers of the potential pandemic nor alerted their populations to those dangers (for recent overviews see Lazzari and Stöhr 2004; Ferguson *et al.* 2006).

Nevertheless, despite recurrent communicable disease the trend towards the greater global burden of noncommunicable disease is clear. In all of the six World Health Organization (WHO) regions except the African region, noncommunicable diseases are more frequent as causes of death than communicable diseases, with a higher cost to poorer populations than to their more wealthy counterparts (Beaglehole and Yach 2003; Yach *et al.* 2005). These trends are predicted to continue so that by 2020 ischaemic heart disease and stroke are expected to be two of the three leading causes of death worldwide. Already seven out of the ten leading causes of death and eight out of the ten leading causes of disability are from noncommunicable sources (WHO 2003). Moreover, the risk factors accounting for these disease patterns are not only well known, they are also all modifiable through coordinated social interventions to tackle what is sometimes referred to as the tobacco and diet/physical activity-related complex of risks (Yach *et al.* 2005). The rapid globalization of the world economy has meant that these disease patterns are fast changing to low- and middle-income countries, with increases in tobacco-, food- and alcohol-related deaths (Beaglehole and Yach 2003) as global manufacturers and distributors take advantage of the marketing opportunities opened up to them in countries that have not yet built effective legal and policy measures to protect the health of their populations. The primary causes of death and disability are now a factor of social and political agency within the control of societies, with effective civil and public health action. In this sense the epidemiological transition can be seen as a change from the primacy of material constraints to social constraints as the limiting condition on health and the quality of human life (Wilkinson 1994), leading some to question why it is that the epidemiological transition has not been accompanied by a matching social transition to greater equality in health between social groups (for a discussion of a failed social transition and its implications, see Chapter 4).

The nutrition transition

Space does not allow an exploration of the impact of these changes on the politics of health through examining individually alcohol, tobacco, food and exercise (see Chapters 10 and 17 for further consideration of the management of tobacco and its risks to health). A brief consideration of food will suffice to reveal the pattern. A seminal study of global food availability, using data between 1962 and 1994, revealed that the traditional relationship between household income and fat consumption has been broken. The global production of cheap oils, fats and sweeteners has changed the diets of people, with dramatic health effects (Drewnowski and Popkin 1997). Although it has long been acknowledged that there is an inverse ratio between obesity and socioeconomic status in high-income countries (Ball and Crawford 2005) it had been assumed that obesity in low- and middle-income countries tended to be a problem for higher socioeconomic groups. However, in middle-income countries obesity is shifting to lower income groups as wealth increases, particularly with women, causing high costs to health services (Monteiro et al. 2004). In the case of China, for example, a recent study (Popkin et al. 2006) revealed that the indirect costs to the country of obesity and changing dietary and exercise patterns was far higher than the direct medical costs. These were estimated to be 3.58 per cent of gross national product (GNP) in 2000 and are projected to rise to 8.73 per cent of GNP by 2025. The WHO has been proactive in attempting to form a global alliance of interested parties to manage the risk of the food transition to health (World Health Assembly 2004), a form of global public health policy and governance as novel and important as its attempts to manage tobacco through the Framework Convention on Tobacco Control (Roemer et al. 2005; for discussion of the policy significance of the Convention see Chapters 10 and 17).

Interventions to manage the health consequences of these trends are strategically dependent on communications, the effective dissemination of independent and rigorous research and alliances for action (Garman 2005). It is disconcerting, therefore, to discover that all three areas of this kind of intervention are being endangered by vested interest. The way in which the tobacco industry for over 40 years is said to have systematically distorted research evidence, compromised the independence of university research and influenced independent health and academic advisory bodies is well documented (Hirschorn 2000; Cohen 2001; Turcotte 2003; see also Chapter 10). The manner in which the food industry attempts the same kind of strategies is only now becoming clear (Ebbeling et al. 2002; Nestle 2003; Cannon 2005). This is perhaps not surprising since food manufacturers and distributors find themselves in contention with public health interest in ways comparable to the tobacco interests of a generation ago. Another reason is that tobacco manufacturers, such as Philip Morris, can be food manufacturers also or might utilize the same kind of lobbying and advertising connections that fund research organizations (Jarlbro 2001; Monbiot 2006). But perhaps there is another and more powerful force at work here. As neoliberal strategies opened up global competition in the last decades of the twentieth century so the boundaries of the public domain supporting the idea of independent scientific research within a neutral academic environment have come increasingly under threat. It is interesting that at the time the senior manager of policy communication within one of the oldest and most prestigious UK scientific bodies, the Royal Society, has written to Exxonmobil (image.guardian.co.uk/sys-files/Guardian/documents/2006/) asking it not to fund organizations that systematically and consciously misrepresent the science of climate change, a series of books (Kassirer 2004; Krimsky 2004; Angell 2005; Washburn 2005) and articles (Davidoff *et al.* 2001; Lexchin *et al.* 2003; Sackett and Oxman 2003; Horton 2004; Smith 2005; Pringle 2006) are emerging that alert the world to the dangerously dominant role that biotechnical, pharmaceutical, food and agricultural companies are playing in the research organizations, scientific journals, universities and pressure groups that shape government health policy.

References

Albala, C. and Vio, F. (1995) Epidemiological transition in Latin America: the case of Chile, *Public Health*, 109(6): 431–42.

Angell, M. (2005) *The Truth About Drug Companies: How they Deceive Us and What to Do About it*. New York: Random House.

Ball, K. and Crawford, D. (2005) Socioeconomic status and weight change in adults: a review, *Social Science and Medicine*, 60(9): 1987–2010.

Barrett, R., Kuzawa, C.W., McDade, T. and Armelagos, G.J. (1998) Emerging and re-emerging infectious diseases: the third epidemiological transition, *Annual Review of Anthropology*, 27: 247–71.

Beaglehole, R. and Yach, D. (2003) Globalisation and the prevention and control of non-communicable disease. the neglected chronic diseases of adults, *The Lancet*, 362(9387): 903–8.

Caldwell, J.C. (1993) Health transition: the cultural, social and behavioural determinants of health in the Third World, *Social Science and Medicine*, 36(2): 125–35.

Cannon, G. (2005) Why the Bush administration and the global sugar industry are determined to demolish the 2004 WHO global strategy on diet, physical activity and health, *Public Health Nutrition*, 7(3): 369–80.

Chesnais, J.C. (1992) *The Demographic Transition: Stages, Patterns and Economic Implications*. Oxford: Clarendon Press.

Cohen, J.E. (2001) Universities and tobacco money, *British Medical Journal*, 323: 1–2.

Coleman, D. (2000) Population and the family, in A.H. Halsey, and J. Webb, (eds) *Twentieth Century British Social Trends*. Basingstoke: Macmillan.

Davidoff, F., DeAngelis, C.D., Drazen, J.M., Hoey, J. and Hojgaard, L. (2001) Sponsorship, authorship, and accountability, *The Lancet*, 358: 854–6.

DoH (Department of Health) (2004) *Choosing Health: Making Healthier Choices Easier*. London: HMSO.

Drewnowski, A. and Popkin, B.M. (1997) The nutrition transition: new trends in the global diet, *Nutrition Review*, 55(2): 31–43.

Ebbeling, C.A., Pawlak, D.B. and Ludwig, D.S. (2002) Childhood obesity: public health crisis, common sense cure, *The Lancet*, 360(9331): 473–82.

Ferguson, N.M., Cummings, D.A., Fraser, C., Cajka, J.C., Cooley, P.C. and Burke D.S. (2006) Strategies for mitigating an influenza pandemic, *Nature*, 442(7101): 448–52.

GAD (Government Actuary's Department) (2005) *Migration and Population Growth*, www.gad.gov.uk/Population/2004/methodology/mignote.htm.

Gage, T.B. (1993) The decline in mortality in England and Wales, 1861–1964: decomposition by cause of death and components of mortality, *Population Studies*, 49(1): 47–66.

Garman, S. (2005) The social context of health promotion in a globalising world, in A. Scriven, and S. Garman (eds) *Promoting Health: Global Perspectives*. Basingstoke: Palgrave Macmillan.

GCIM (Global Commission on International Migration) (2005) *Migration in an Interconnected World: New Directions for Action*, www.gcim.org/en/finalreport.html.

Gillis, J.R., Tilly, L.A. and Levine, D. (eds) (1992) *The European Experience of Declining Fertility 1850–1970: The Quiet Revolution*. Oxford: Oxford University Press.

Health Canada (2004) www.hc-sc.gc.ca/pphb-dgspsp/cpip-pclcpi.

Hirschorn, N. (2000) Shameful science; four decades of the German tobacco industry's hidden research on smoking and health, *Tobacco Control*, 9: 242–7.

Horton, R. (2004) The dawn of McScience, *New York Review of Books*, 51(4): 7–9.

Hunt, A. (1999) *Governing Morals: A Social History of Moral Regulation*. Cambridge: Cambridge University Press.

James, H. (2001) *The End of Globalization*. Cambridge, MA: Harvard University Press.

Jarlbro, G. (2001) *Children and Advertising: The Players, the Arguments and the Research During the Period 1994–2000*. Stockholm: Swedish Consumer Agency.

Kassirer, J.P. (2004) *On the Take: How Medicine's Complicity with Big Business can Endanger your Health*. New York: Oxford University Press.

Kiernan, K. (2004) Cohabitation and divorce across nations and generations, in P.L. Chase-Lansdale, K. Kiernan and R.J. Friedman (eds) *Human Development Across Lives and Generations: The Potential for Change*. Cambridge: Cambridge University Press.

Kirk, D. (1996) Demographic transition theory, *Population Studies*, 50: 361–87.

Kluger, R. (1996) *Ashes to Ashes: America's Hundred Year Cigarette War. The Public Health and the Unabashed Triumph of Philip Morris*. New York: Alfred A. Knopf.

Kotlikoff, L.J. and Raffelhuschen, B. (1999) Generational accounting around the globe, *The American Economic Review*, 89(2): 161–6.

Krimsky, S. (2004) *Science in the Private Interest: Has the Lure of Profits Corrupted Biomedical Research?* Lanham, MD: Rowman & Littlefield.

Lazzari, S. and Stöhr, K. (2004) Avian influenza and influenza pandemics, *Bulletin of the World Health Organization*, 82(4): 242.

Lexchin J., Bero, L.A., Djulbegovic, B. and Clark, O. (2003) Pharmaceutical industry sponsorship and research outcome and quality, *British Medical Journal*, 326: 1167–70.

MacLehose, L., McKee, M. and Weinberg, J. (2002) Responding to the challenge of communicable disease in Europe, *Science*, 295(5562): 2047–50.

McCarthy, K. (2001) *World Population Shifts: Boom or Doom?* Santa Monica, CA: Rand.

McKee, M. (2005) European health policy: where now? *European Journal of Public Health*, 15(6): 557–8.

Migration Watch (2006) *Migration Trends*. Briefing papers 9.2,15, May.

Monbiot, G. (2006) The tobacco industry duped both academic journals and the media, *Guardian*, 7 February.

Monteiro, C.A., Moura, E.C., Conde, W.L. and Popkin, B.M. (2004) Socioeconomic status and obesity in adult populations of developing countries: a review, *Bulletin of the World Health Organization*, 82(12): 940–6.

NAO (National Audit Office) (2005) *Returning Failed Asylum Seekers*, HC76, session 2005–6. London: The Stationery Office.

Nestle, M. (2003) *Safe Food: Bacteria, Biotechnology, and Bioterrorism*. Berkeley, CA: University of California Press.

ONS (Office for National Statistics) (2006) *Social Trends 36*. London: ONS.

Omran, A.R. (2005) The epidemiologic transition: a theory of the epidemiology of population change, *The Milbank Quarterly*, 83(4): 731–57.

Popkin, B.M., Kim, S., Rusev, E.R., Du, S. and Zizza, C. (2006) Measuring the full economic costs of diet, physical activity and obesity-related chronic diseases, *Obesity Review*, 7(3): 271–93.

Pringle, E. (2006) *Big Pharma Research Racket is Killing People*. www.sierratimes.com/06/06/24/75_7_241_211_29304.htm.

Reuters (2006) Asylum row overshadows Home Office reforms, posted 19 July, www.Reuters.Co.UK/news.

Roemer, J.D., Allyn Taylor, J.S.D. and Lariviere, J. (2005) Origins of the WHO Framework convention on Tobacco Control, *American Journal of Public Health*, 95(6): 936–8.

Sackett, D.L. and Oxman, A.D. (2003) HARLOT plc: an amalgamation of the world's two oldest professions, *British Medical Journal*, 327: 1442–5.

Salomon, J.A. and Murray, C.J. (2002) The epidemiologic transition revisited: compositional models for causes of death by age and sex, *Population and Development Review*, 28(2): 205–28.

Schofield, R., Reher, D. and Bideau, A. (eds) (1991) *The Decline of Mortality in Europe*. Oxford: Oxford University Press.

Shorter, E. (1983) *A History of Women's Bodies*. Harmondsworth: Penguin.

Smith, R. (2005) Medical journals are an extension of the marketing arm of pharmaceutical companies, *PLoS Medicine*, 2(5): e138.

Stolnitz, G.J. (ed.) (1994) *Social Aspects and Country Reviews of Population Aging: Europe and North America*. United Nations Economic Commission for Europe, Economic Studies No. 6. Geneva: United Nations.

Turcotte, F. (2003) Why universities should stay away from tobacco money, *Drug and Alcohol Review*, 22: 107–8.

Waite, L. and Gallagher, M. (2000) *The Case for Marriage*. New York: Doubleday.

Washburn, J. (2005) *University, Inc: The Corporate Corruption of Higher Education*. New York: Basic Books.

WHO (2003) *World Health Report 2003: Shaping the Future*. Geneva: WHO.

Wilkinson, R.G. (1994) The epidemiological transition: from material scarcity to social disadvantage? *Daedalus*, 123: 61–77.

World Health Assembly (2004) *Global Strategy on Diet, Physical Activity and Health*. Geneva: WHO.

Yach, D., Beaglehole, R. and Hawkes, C. (2005) Globalisation and noncommunicable diseases, in A. Scriven, and S. Garman (eds) *Promoting Health: Global Perspectives*. Basingstoke: Palgrave Macmillan.

4 Social patterning of health behaviours

Graham Scambler and Sasha Scambler

There are stark inequalities in life expectancy between nation states, and in the last decade these inequalities have increased. The expectation of life at birth in high-income countries is 20 years longer than in low-income countries, of which two-thirds of the population is in south Asia, and one-third in sub-Saharan Africa (Therborn 2006: 20–1). The newborn in high-income countries, comprising 15 per cent of the world's population of newborn, enjoy a life expectancy approximately 11 years longer than average compared to those born in low-income countries with life expectations 9 years shorter than the human average.

Although country differences in life expectancy had diminished for 40 years, during the 1990s this trend was halted and divergence displaced convergence (Moser *et al.* 2005). Technically, the dispersion measure of mortality increased from 1950 to 2000, but this was due in large part to the fact that 24 countries experienced falling life expectancies in the 1990s; 16 of the 24 were in sub-Saharan Africa and 6 in the former Soviet Union (for a discussion of the dispersion index of mortality, see Moser *et al.* 2005; for a comparison with the alternative slope measure of inequality, see Dorling *et al.* 2006).

Over the last century life expectancy has increased by between two and three decades in high-income countries. Initially, infant and child mortality fell dramatically, precipitating a decline in birth rates, a phenomenon known as the demographic transition, followed by a series of epidemiological transitions. Infectious diseases yielded to chronic conditions like circulatory disease and cancer, and in the high-income countries of western Europe there is evidence of a decline in chronic disease mortality rates since the 1970s (for further discussion of both the demographic and epidemiological transitions, see Chapter 3). However, there has been no corresponding sociological transition (Vagero 2006); while absolute differences between the social classes have reduced within the UK, remarkably the relative mortality ratio is almost exactly the same at the end as at the beginning of this period.

In Britain, Michael Marmot and his colleagues have been the principal documenters of this relative mortality ratio and the inertia it reflects. In a series of pioneering socio-epidemiological studies they have repeatedly shown what they describe as a social gradient, indicating that the lower the occupational class or socioeconomic group (SEG) or socioeconomic status (SES), the greater the risk of premature death (Marmot 2004, 2006). People on the lower rungs of the social or occupational ladder typically run at least twice the risk of serious illness and premature death as those near the top. Moreover, within the ranks of middle class office personnel, lower-ranking staff experience more disease and earlier death than higher-ranking staff (Wilkinson and Marmot 2003). Figure 4.1, which summarizes occupational class differences in life expectancy for England and Wales, 1997–9, will be taken here to epitomize data on the social gradient. Indeed, there are indications that the social gradient may be steeper now than a generation ago (Shaw *et al.* 1999).

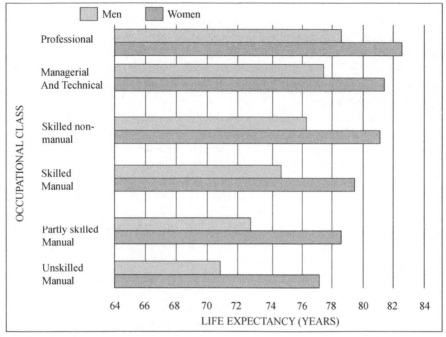

Figure 4.1 Life expectancy of men and women, England and Wales, 1997–9
Source: CSDH (2005)

Wilkinson and Marmot (2003: 10) suggest the following by way of a summary of the current explanation: that both material and psychosocial causes and their effects contribute to these differences; that these effects include most diseases and most causes of death; that disadvantage has many forms such as fewer family assets, poorer education during adolescence, insecure employment, hazardous or dead end jobs, poor housing, difficult family circumstances and inadequate retirement pensions; that the disadvantages tend to concentrate among the same people; and the effects on health accumulate through life (for strategies of intervention designed to ameliorate such structured health inequalities see Chapters 12 and 13; for initiatives focused on neighbourhood, workplace and housing see Chapters 14, 15 and 18 respectively; for city strategies, see Chapter 16).

Mackenbach (2006: 31) usefully divides factors known to bear on health inequalities into three categories: material factors, psychosocial factors and lifestyle factors. Although there is variation between European Union (EU) countries, the tendency for health behaviours conducive to morbidity and premature mortality to cluster in the lower social echelons has been well established.

Models of health inequality

It is one thing to list factors causally pertinent to the social gradient, and then to categorize them, and another to develop models or theories to account for or explain it. Here there might, and arguably should, be disciplinary differences. The public health physician or advocate is likely to prioritize pragmatic interventions, for example to reduce health inequalities, and here the positivistic character of epidemiological research comes to the fore: it is predictive efficiency that matters, at least in the short term. For other disciplines, from the life and clinical to the behavioural and social sciences, predicting is not, or should not be, regarded positivistically as equivalent to or, worse, synonymous with, explaining.

In a discussion paper for the newly established and public health-oriented Commission on Social Determinants of Health, Solar and Irwin (2005) summarize four of the many models that have been advanced to account for the social gradient. Whitehead and Dahlgren's (1991) model of layered influences attempts to demonstrate how social inequalities in health are the product of interactions between different levels, or layers, of causal conditions, ranging from individuals at one end of the spectrum to general socioeconomic, cultural and environmental conditions at the other. Individuals are located at the centre of this five-layer model, each endowed with age, sex and genetic factors that influence their health potential. Moving outwards, the next layer represents personal behaviours and lifestyles. As has been noted above, individuals in disadvantaged circumstances tend to exhibit a higher prevalence of risky behaviours, like smoking, while also facing greater financial barriers to opting for healthier lifestyles. Social and community influences are positioned on the third layer. These feature social networks and other systems of support, both informal and formal. The penultimate layer consists of factors relating to living and working conditions, the supply of goods, and access to pivotal facilities and services. Finally, and overarching all other levels or layers, are the economic, cultural and environmental properties of society as a whole. Included here are: the economic profile of the nation state, labour market conditions and pervasive cultural norms.

The social stratification and disease production model (Diderichsen *et al.* 1998 cited by Solar and Irwin 2005) emphasizes how an individual's social position sets parameters for health opportunities. The mechanisms that lead to such social positioning are the structures of society that generate and distribute power, wealth and risk such as the education system, labour policies, cultural norms and political institutions. An individual's social position, in its turn, helps determine exposure to health-damaging circumstances, vulnerability and the impact of ill health over time.

The selection and causation model (Mackenbach 1994 cited by Solar and Irwin 2005) puts the accent on the mechanisms that generate health inequalities, and features both selection and causation. Reference is made, first, to the selection processes that represent the effects of ill health in adulthood on both occupational class and the nature and degree of ill health through adult phases of the life course. The causation mechanism, second, is represented by three groups of risk factors that mediate between socio-economic position and ill health: material or structural/environmental, psychosocial and lifestyle factors. Childhood environment, cultural and psychological factors are also incorporated in the model in recognition of their contribution to inequalities in health through a mix of selection and causation.

Finally, Brunner, Marmot and Wilkinson's model, which occupied a central position in the Acheson report of 1998, emphasizes multiple influences across the life course (Acheson 1998 cited by Solar and Irwin 2005). It was originally devised to connect clinical or curative and public health or preventive orientations to health, but was subsequently modified to accommodate factors that both cause ill health and contribute to health inequalities. The authors claim that the model links social structure to health and disease via material, psychosocial and behavioural pathways. Genetic, early life and cultural factors are also acknowledged as important influences on population health.

What is striking about these models is the extent of their overlap, their easy compatibility with the relevant national and international data and their lack of explanatory ambition or power.

A recent attempt at synthesis (Solar and Irwin 2005) suggests that social and political contexts generate sets of unequal socioeconomic positions, leading to stratified difference by factors such as income, education, professional status, gender and ethnicity. Socioeconomic positions represent both the structural determinants of health inequalities and the specific determinants of health status; they imply differential exposure and vulnerability to factors known to compromise health. These specific determinants of ill health are seen as intermediary determinants. Relevant here are material conditions, like work and housing circumstances; psychosocial conditions, like stressful life events; and behavioural factors, like smoking.

A distinctive feature of this synthetic model is its incorporation of the healthcare system. Solar and Irwin note a feedback effect of health on socioeconomic position, such as when an individual experiences a fall in income because of a work induced disability. They point out that the Department of Health (DoH) in the UK has recommended a more proactive stance in reducing health inequalities by ensuring equitable access to healthcare services and by establishing public health programmes targeted at disadvantaged communities (see also Mackenbach and Gunning-Schepers 1997). They suggest an elaborated model of social determinants of health for the future work of the Commission on Social Determinants of Health deploying the distinction between structural and intermediary determinants (see Figure 4.2).

A great deal of sophisticated investigative work, most of it social epidemiological, has gone into the construction of these models. What models typically do, however, is arrange or rearrange factors known to be causally implicated in a phenomenon like health inequalities without doing much to explain it. Models tend to be heuristic devices, their merits being extrinsic rather than intrinsic. Explanations, on the other hand, necessarily involve the setting out of testable theory.

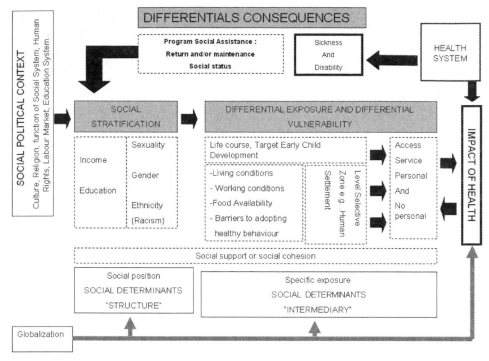

Figure 4.2   Conceptual framework
Source: CSDH (2005: 16)

From models to theories

In an attempt to advance the theory of health inequalities, Wilkinson makes a general case that once societies have negotiated the epidemiological transition and a certain level of gross national product (GNP) per capita is attained, approximately US$5000 at 1996 prices, the principal determinant of level of health status within a nation state is the degree of income inequality (Wilkinson 1996: 3).

With reference to the Organization for Economic Cooperation and Development (OECD) countries, he claims that the degree of income inequality explains about three-quarters of the variation in life expectancy across countries, whereas, by itself, the absolute size of the economic pie, measured by GNP per capita, accounts for less than 10 per cent of the variation (Wilkinson 1992). Not everyone agrees with this relative income hypothesis (see for example Judge 1995), but considerable support for Wilkinson's findings has accumulated in low-, medium- and high-income societies. No less distinctive is his explanation. Following Putnam (1983) he maintains that social cohesion and trust are the mechanisms linking the degree of income inequality with health (for a further introduction to Putnam's work and its influence, see Chapter 6) so that income inequality burdens people with both the effects of low social status and those of poor social affiliations (Wilkinson 2000: 998). There is firm evidence, he believes, that where income differences are more marked, social divisions tend to be exacerbated; levels of trust and strength of community life diminished; rates of social anxiety and chronic stress enhanced; rates of hostility, violence and homicide increased. Moreover there is a propensity for a culture of inequality characterized by a more hostile and less hospitable social environment to develop (Wilkinson 1999a, 1999b). In other words the actual experience of low social status or subordination (Wilkinson 2000: 998–9) is as important as material circumstances in explaining health inequalities.

Wilkinson has been criticized for his measurement of changing national rates of income inequality, his definition of social cohesion and trust, his privileging of psychosocial pathways and, latterly, his willingness to infer from animal to human behaviour (see for example Coburn 2000). His work is important for its positing a plausible and testable theory of health inequalities. Coburn's own contribution arises from his observation that there has been an overwhelming tendency to focus on possible social and psychobiological mechanisms through which social factors might be tied to health at the expense of considering the social causes of inequality and health. These he identifies as the neoliberal economics of market dominance (Coburn 2000: 136–7; see also Muntaner and Lynch 1999). He attributes three assumptions to the new neoliberal order: that markets are the optimally efficient allocators of resources in production and distribution; that societies are composed of individual producers and consumers motivated primarily by material considerations; and that competition is the vehicle for innovations. Economic globalization and neoliberalism, he suggests, are natural bedfellows. Allowing a possible exception in Japan, he contends that the more neoliberal or market oriented the nation state, the greater the income inequality within its borders, the higher the level of social fragmentation and the lower the social cohesion and trust.

In a recent paper Coburn posits a more explicitly class-based or class welfare regime model, arguing that global political and economic trends have increased the power of business classes at the expense of the working classes (Coburn 2004; see also Scambler and Higgs 2001). He argues that international pressures towards neoliberal doctrines and policies have been differentially resisted by nation states, largely because of their differing historical and institutional structures; that social epidemiological research indicates that neoliberalism is associated with greater income inequalities, both nationally and internationally. Countries with more social democratic welfare regimes, such as Finland, Sweden and Norway, have better health than those with more markedly neoliberal regimes, namely the USA and the UK. Coburn's (2004: 44–5) model is epitomized in Figure 4.3.

Most previous analyses, he suggests, link factors in C with health or wellbeing (D), while his model advances the causal explanation by including the determinants A and B.

Consonant with Coburn's revised position, Scambler and Higgs (1999, 2001) stress the political significance of neoliberalism because of its potential to rationalize class action. They adopt a neo Marxist theoretical stance based on critical realism (see also Forbes and Wainwright 2001) by suggesting that economic relations of class have in fact grown in causal efficacy relative to state relations of command in the context of the nation state during the era of what has variously been called global or disorganized capitalism dating from the early to mid-1970s to the present.

Scambler (2001, 2002), following Clement and Myles (1997), identifies what he calls the capitalist executive, as strategic in his analysis; a construct which provides the currency for a 'greedy bastards hypothesis' (GBH). This asserts that Britain's widening health

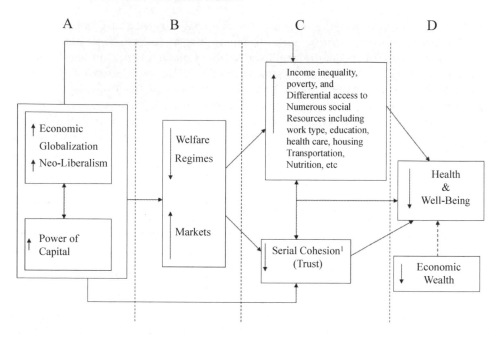

Figure 4.3   The class/welfare regime model
Source: Coburn (2004: 44)

inequalities might reasonably be regarded as the largely unintended consequence of the ever adaptive behaviours of its weakly globalized power elite, informed by the increasingly irresistible, voracious and strategic appetites of core members of its strongly globalized capitalist executive. Documentation of greed is readily available. Within the UK, for example, some 2000 people in the City of London received bonuses of at least £1 million in 2000 while in 2004, 230 FTSE 100 company directors were paid more than £1 million (see Lansley 2006). Moreover rewards are often earned by containing or cutting labour costs and, more circuitously, by limiting social transfers (Gupta 2002).

At the kernel of the GBH is the reinvigoration of class relations relative to those of command. It is an issue of social structure. It is entirely plausible to insist that the strategic decision making conducted by a small, focused core alliance is a vital, direct and intended determinant of the changing pattern of labour and of income and social transfers in Britain. An unintended consequence is enduring and widening health inequalities. In other words, the destandardization of work and the new inequality, as well as derivative processes like the new individualization, and therefore the widening of health inequalities, have their genesis in the adaptive behaviours of those in power (Scambler 2002). The confinement of wealth and power to largely unexamined boxes in many social epidemiological and even sociological models of health inequalities is incongruous enough to warrant empirical investigation in its own right (Scambler 1996).

It is instructive to compare this position with that of Marmot. Marmot's central contention is that for people above a certain threshold of material wellbeing another kind of wellbeing is central, namely autonomy. He suggests that inequalities in the degree to which people control their lives are strategic to health and underpin the status syndrome (Marmot 2004: 2). He further suggests that while all societies are unequal, they differ widely in the gradient of their health inequalities, and that the latter are demonstrably related to the opportunities available for people to control their lives (Marmot 2004: 24). Some determinants of health can be seen to act independently of social position. While improvement in environment and health behaviours can benefit the health of all regardless of social status, these determinants do not explain the social gradient. The putative causal roles of autonomy and social participation came to light precisely because the gradient could not be centrally attributed predominantly to differences in smoking, diet and other aspects of lifestyle.

Health behaviours: a critical realist framework

The philosophy of critical realism developed by Roy Bhaskar was in many respects intended to be an extension of the work of Marx. It has been explicated elsewhere (Scambler 2002) and only an abbreviated summary will be attempted here. It is a perspective that recognizes that the events people experience by means of empirical awareness and examination are indebted to the causal powers of deep or real structures. This is accepted readily enough in the natural and life sciences but meets resistance when the behavioural or social sciences are discussed. Scientific research depends on the successful identification of the relatively enduring structures or generative mechanisms that must exist for the events to occur. However, in complex open systems like the social worlds humans inhabit, there is never a one-to-one correspondence between any given structure, such as relations of class, command, status, gender, ethnicity or age, and events to be explained.

Figure 4.4 summarizes the structural premises underlying the GBH. It claims that with the switch from organized to disorganized capitalism through the 1970s a shift in the nature of the logic of the regime of capital accumulation, articulated in relations of class, has occasioned a requisite shift in the nature of the mode of regulation, articulated in relations of command, in the figuration of the British nation state. The result has been a ceding of ground by relations of command to those of class. The GBH is an epiphenomenon of this reinvigoration of class.

In similar vein to Coburn, it is argued here that class relations need to be distinguished from occupational class and social status categories and that the former represent the single most significant structure or generative mechanism for explaining health inequalities (for a different approach to the significance of social class for health, see Chapter 5). It is a transcendental argument: this must be the case given what is known about the properties and extent of health inequalities but how can this thesis be defended, and what kind of research programme might it generate?

There is a strong case for resisting the common view that there are discrete, identifiable pathways connecting class relations and class categories via prescribed routes, such as those of low social cohesion, to health outcomes (for measurements linking social cohesion to health, see Chapter 6). The evidence suggests it is much more likely that there are innumerable, different and changing routes to these same end points. Nor does Krieger's (1994) seductive notion of a web appear especially salutary since concepts of pathways and webs smack of neo-positivism, with all its philosophical baggage.

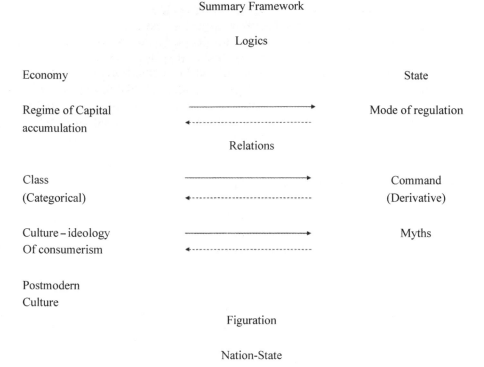

Figure 4.4   Summary framework

It might be fruitful to think less in terms of trying to identify specific pathways or webs by means of multivariate analyses, and more in terms of elucidating those capital or asset flows pertinent to health by means of research in a critical realist mode. The concept of asset flows builds on a wealth of previous investigations, some represented here, but most notably on the significance of material factors and of time and the life course; relations of class systematically affect the asset flows to individuals of different types of assets with potential to impact on health and longevity. These flows are typically variable and almost certainly of special salience at critical periods of the life course.

At least six types of asset flow are known to be important for health and longevity. The flow of biological or body assets can be affected by class relations even prior to birth. Low income families, for example, are more likely to produce babies of low birth weight (Power *et al.* 1996); and low birth weight babies carry an increased risk of chronic disease in childhood, possibly through biological programming (Barker 1992). Psychological assets yield a generalized capacity to cope, extending to what Rutter (1985) once described as resilience in the face of adversity (for a further discussion of resilience, class and health, see Chapter 5). In many respects, the vulnerability factors that Brown and Harris (1978) found reduced working class women's capacity to cope with categories of life event of causal import for episodes of clinical depression are class-induced interruptions to the flow of psychological assets. Social assets have come to assume pride of place in many accounts of health inequalities and feature strongly in those of Wilkinson and Marmot. The terms social assets or social capital refer to aspects of social integration, networks and support (for a detailed discussion of social capital including its measurement, see Chapter 6). The fact that it has proved politically expedient to latch onto a lack of social capital as a cause of health inequalities, and that measures of social capital have betrayed a middle class bias favouring, say, church attendance over gang membership (Muntaner *et al.* 1999), should not occasion its neglect. Cultural assets or cultural capital are generated initially through processes of primary socialization and go on to encompass formal educational opportunities and attainment. Class-related early arrests to the flow of cultural assets can have long term ramifications for employment, income levels and therefore health (Plesis 2000). Area-based studies have established the salience for health also of spatial assets. There is clear evidence that areas of high mortality tend to be areas with high rates of net emigration; and it tends to be the better qualified and more affluent who exercise the option to leave (Shaw *et al.* 1999).

There exist also the strategically significant material assets. There may be a ready interaction between asset flows, but it is self evidently the case both that the flow of material assets is fundamental and an influence on all others. For example, if the flow of material assets dries up, the flow of spatial assets must surely follow suit. It is this flow that is most directly responsive to class relations. Marmot's focus on status syndrome, substituting for time-honoured sociological notions like relative deprivation and reference groups, merely reinforces this point.

An advantage of the concept of capital or asset flows is the implicit recognition that assets can vary over time and their possession is a matter of degree. The concept allows for the possibility that a strong asset flow will compensate for another weaker one: a reduced biological asset flow might be compensated for by a strong psychological asset flow, or an arrest in the flow of material assets by strong flows of social or cultural assets.

The empirical investigation of variable and interactive asset flows and their health effects, however, requires a more imaginative philosophy and methodology than those associated with neopositivism. Asset flows cannot readily be reduced to a set of indicators or variables. Critical realists advocate alternative methodologies to the inductive and deductive inference used in social epidemiology and positivist sociology. They commend instead retroduction in quantitative and abduction in qualitative research. Both retroduction and abduction acknowledge that the effects of beneath the surface structures or generative mechanisms, like class relations, cannot simply be read in on the surface events. This is because events tend to be both unsynchronized with the mechanisms that govern them and determined by various, perhaps countervailing, influences (Lawson 1997: 22). In other words, the theoretical objects of sociological inquiry, like relations of class, status or gender, only manifest themselves in open systems where constant event patterns or regularities of the kind pursued through variable analysis rarely, if ever, obtain.

Lawson (1997: 24) refers to retroduction as a kind of 'as if' reasoning: moving from the conception of some phenomenon of interest to a structure or condition that is, at least in part, responsible for its existence. Abduction is similarly geared to the identification of structures or mechanisms, but involves a process of inference from lay or first order accounts of events to sociological or second order accounts of structures or mechanisms (Blaikie 1993). Bhaskar (1978) characterizes critical realist science in terms of a threefold process. A phenomenon, such as health inequalities in a particular figuration, is identified. Explanations based on the postulated existence of a generative mechanism, such as class relations, are constructed and empirically tested. This mechanism then becomes the phenomenon to be explained, and so on. Thus, realist science involves a process of description, explanation and redescription, in which layers of reality are continually exposed. It is important to add that although constant event patterns or invariant regularities may not obtain in open systems, partial regularities do. Lawson (1997: 204) labels these as demi regularities.

A recent review of work on tackling health inequalities (Asthana and Halliday 2006: 30) is supportive both of the emphasis, reiterated here, on the structural bases of health inequalities, made manifest in wealth and power, and of the deployment of the concept of capital or asset flows as the media of enactment of relations of class. However, it is not convinced that the approach offered here adds much either to sociological under-standing or as a guide to policy since it does little more than restate the links between causal factors at an individual level while acknowledging the inevitable vagueness about identifying the structural factors in which they are located. These points about the re-lations of the individual to social structures as well as the implications for policy will now be considered.

Health behaviours conventionally refer to risky behaviours like smoking, binge drinking, consuming fast foods and sedentary habits. Risky though these behaviours are, the politically convenient payoffs of both the easy attribution of individual responsi-bility, and also the distancing of government responsibility, cannot be ignored. It has become ever clearer since the publication of the UK Black Report in 1980 that health behaviours, like all behaviours, are socially structured, if not structurally determined (Asthana and Halliday 2006). People in low income families do not show a greater pro-pensity to smoke because they are stupid or irresponsible (Graham 1995). Moreover there is an unequivocal case for identifying another category of behaviours, epitomized in those of the GBs of the GBH, as health behaviours.

Since leaders in both private- and public-sector institutions drive or sign up to social change consonant with their class based vested interests, their behaviours might rea-sonably be characterized as health behaviours. The trend for managers to increase their pay and pensions and attract recognition in honours lists is a consequence of downsizing workforces, replacing permanent by part time or contract workers, reducing work au-tonomy in favour of managerial control, outsourcing and ending final salary pension schemes for new and even existing workers. By doing so they deleteriously affect the health and longevity of the working class and its 'displaced segment' (Scambler and Higgs 1999) or underclass. Nor can the GBs claim a lack of reflexivity in the reflexive moder-nization of disorganized capitalism (Beck et al. 1994; Scambler 2001).

It is of course less than politically expedient to attribute a more telling health-related or structured agency to the director of a FTSE 100 company than to an unemployed bricklayer. It might be objected too that the former is pivotal for wealth creation, and therefore for the medium to long term improvement in population health some prices are worth paying. But Wilkinson's linkage of income inequalities with health inequalities amounts to more than a qualification. Two major theses merit further investigation. The first is that social class, through the health behaviours of core members of the capitalist executive, opens or shuts the valves that control capital or asset flows most salient for health and longevity. Other social structures can open or close these same valves, but class relations are predominant in the figuration of the nation state (Scambler 2002).

Second, class based closure of the valves controlling the flow of material assets in the critical juncture of infancy and early childhood is especially telling for general health in both early and later phases of the life course (see Asthana and Halliday 2006: 107–53 for a review of the evidence).

Policy: tackling health inequalities

Public health, with its disciplinary base in epidemiology, is appropriately oriented to policies to reduce health inequalities (for an assessment of the effectiveness of policy, see Chapter 11). To this end the neopositivist accent on prediction is apt. Sociologists adjoined to this same enterprise might reasonably follow suit: policy sociology is an indispensable branch of the discipline. However, policy sociology can only too readily be coopted to fit external agendas (Burawoy 2005). Professional sociology underwrites not only the application of disciplinary perspectives and research to address and help solve policy issues, but also a more critical sociology of, for example, the formation, implementation and political rationales for policy. Any independent critical sociology must recognize that the announcement and even enactment of policies to reduce health inequalities are likely to serve quite other, more political functions, like securing public legitimacy. In this sense there is no contradiction in asserting that programmes purporting to tackle health inequalities in the UK can be entirely and knowingly consistent with the widening gap in health inequalities (Shaw *et al.* 1999). To denounce politicians as cynical and manipulative is simplistic. Nevertheless it is a vital task confronting public sociology to call the political executive to account, not least for their injurious health behaviours. (This is not to say that increasing income and health inequalities cannot be ameliorated by policy initiatives aimed at the most vulnerable. For the success of such initiatives, see in particular Chapters 11, 12 and 13.)

It should perhaps be reiterated here that this is not a critique of public health specialists whose work is dedicated to policy revision nor of the lobbying for government-sponsored interventions that it heralds (see Siegrist and Marmot 2006). The point is that medical sociology cannot stop at policy sociology. If it does, then it has been tamed, a genuine hazard against the background of the insidious commodification of intellectual endeavour in disorganized capitalism (Scambler 1996). What is also required is a critical mass of critical and public sociologists.

References

Asthana, S. and Halliday, J. (2006) *What Works in Tackling Health Inequalities? Pathways, Policies and Practice Through the Lifecourse*. Bristol: The Policy Press.

Barker, D. (1992) *Foetal and Infant Origins of Adult Disease*. London: BMJ.

Beck, U., Giddens, A. and Lash, S. (1994) *Reflexive Modernization: Politics, Tradition and Aesthetics in the Modern Social Order*. Cambridge: Polity Press.

Bhaskar, R. (1978) *The Realist Theory of Science*, 2nd edn. Brighton: Harvester Wheatsheaf.

Blaikie, N. (1993) *Approaches to Social Enquiry*. Cambridge: Polity Press.

Brown, G. and Harris, T. (1978) *Social Origins of Depression*. London: Tavistock.

Burawoy, T. (2005) The critical turn to public sociology, *Critical Sociology*, 31(3): 313–26.

Clement, W. and Myles, J. (1997) *Relations of Ruling: Class and Gender in Postindustrial Societies*. Montreal: McGill-Queen's University Press.

Coburn, D. (2000) Income inequality, social cohesion and the health status of populations: the role of neo-liberalism, *Social Science and Medicine*, 51: 135–46.

Coburn, D. (2004) Beyond the income inequality hypothesis: class, neo-liberalism, and health inequalities, *Social Science and Medicine*, 58: 41–56.

CSDH (Commission on Social Determinants of Health) (2005) *Towards a Conceptual Framework for Analysis and Action on the Social Determinants of Health*, www.who.int/social_determinants/resources/framework.pdf.

Dorling, D., Shaw, M. and Davey Smith, G. (2006) Global inequality and life expectancy due to AIDS, *British Medical Journal*, 332: 662–4.

Forbes, A. and Wainwright, S. (2001) On the methodological, theoretical and philosophical context of health inequalities research, *Social Science and Medicine*, 51: 801–16.

Graham, H. (1995) Cigarette smoking: a light on gender and class inequality in Britain, *Journal of Social Policy*, 24: 509–27.

Gupta, S. (2002) *Corporate Capitalism and Political Philosophy*. London: Pluto Press.

Judge, K. (1995) Income distribution and life expectancy: a critical appraisal, *British Medical Journal*, 311: 1282–5.

Krieger, N. (1994) Epidemiology and the web of causation: has anyone seen the spider? *Social Science and Medicine*, 39: 887–903.

Lansley, S. (2006) *Rich Britain: The Rise and Rise of the 'New' Super-Wealthy*. London: Politicos.

Lawson, T. (1997) *Economics and Reality*. London: Routledge.

Mackenbach, J. (2006) *Health Inequalities: Europe in Profile*. London: EU.

Mackenbach, J. and Gunning-Schepers, L. (1997) How should interventions to reduce inequalities in health be evaluated? *Journal of Epidemiology and Community Health*, 51: 359–64.

Marmot, M. (2004) *Status Syndrome: How Your Social Standing Directly Affects Your Health and Life Expectancy*. London: Bloomsbury.

Marmot, M. (2006) *Social Determinants of Health Inequalities*. Geneva: WHO.

Moser, K., Leon, D. and Shkolnikov, V. (2005) World mortality 1950–2000: divergence replaces convergence from the late 1980s, *Bulletin of the World Health Organization*, 83: 202–9.

Muntaner, C. and Lynch, J. (1999) Income inequality, social cohesion, and class relations: a critique of Wilkinson's neo-Durkheimian research programme, *International Journal of Health Services*, 29: 59–81.

Muntaner, C., Lynch, J. and Oates, G. (1999) The social class determinants of income inequality and social cohesion, *International Journal of Health Services*, 29: 699–732.

Plesis, I. (2000) Educational inequalities and Education Action Zones, in C. Pantazis and D. Gordon (eds) *Tackling Inequalities: Where are We Now and What Can be Done?* Bristol: The Policy Press.

Power, C., Bartley, M., Blane, D. and Davey Smith, G. (1996) Birthweight and later social circumstances in men and women, in D. Blane, E. Brunner and R. Wilkinson (eds) *Health and Social Organization*. London: Routledge.

Putnam, R. (1983) *Making Democracy Work: Civic Traditions in Modern Italy*. Princeton, NJ: Princeton University Press.

Rutter, M. (1985) Resilience in the face of adversity, *British Journal of Psychiatry*, 147: 598–611.

Scambler, G. (1996) The 'project of modernity' and the parameters for a critical sociology: an argument with illustrations from medical sociology, *Sociology*, 30: 567–81.

Scambler, G. (2001) Class, power and the durability of health inequalities, in G. Scambler (ed.) *Habermas, Critical Theory and Health*. London: Routledge.

Scambler, G. (2002) *Health and Social Change: A Critical Theory*. Buckingham: Open University Press.

Scambler, G. and Higgs, P. (1999) Stratification, class and health: class relations and health inequalities in high modernity, *Sociology*, 33: 275–96.

Scambler, G. and Higgs, P. (2001) 'The dog that didn't bark': taking class seriously in the health inequalities debate, *Social Science and Medicine*, 52: 157–9.

Shaw, M., Dorling, D., Gordon, D. and Davey Smith, G. (1999) *The Widening Gap: Health Inequalities and Policy in Britain*. Bristol: The Policy Press.

Siegrist, J. and Marmot, M. (eds) (2006) *Social Inequalities in Health: New Evidence and Policy Implications*. Oxford: Oxford University Press.

Solar, O. and Irwin, A. (2005) *Towards a Conceptual Framework for Analysis and Action on the Social Determinants of Health*. Geneva: WHO.

Therborn, G. (2006) Meaning, mechanisms, patterns, and forces: an introduction, in G. Therborn, (ed.) *Inequalities of the World: New Theoretical Frameworks, Multiple Empirical Approaches*. London: Verso.

Vagero, D. (2006) Do health inequalities persist in the new global order? A European perspective, in G. Therborn (ed.) *Inequalities of the World: New Theoretical Frameworks, Multiple Empirical Approaches*. London: Verso.

Whitehead, M. and Dahlgren, G. (1991) What can be done about inequalities in health? *The Lancet*, 338(8778): 1337.

Wilkinson, R. (1992) Income distribution and life expectancy, *British Medical Journal*, 304: 165–8.

Wilkinson, R. (1996) *Unhealthy Societies: The Afflictions of Inequality*. London: Routledge.

Wilkinson, R. (1999a) Income inequality, social cohesion and health: clarifying the theory – a reply to Muntaner and Lynch, *International Journal of Health Services*, 29: 525–43.

Wilkinson, R. (1999b) The culture of inequality, in B. Kawachi, B. Kennedy, and R. Wilkinson, (eds) *Income Inequality and Health: The Society and Population Health Reader*, Vol. 1. New York: New Press.

Wilkinson, R. (2000) Deeper than neo-liberalism: a reply to David Coburn, *Social Science and Medicine*, 51: 997–1000.

Wilkinson, R. and Marmot, M. (eds) (2003) *Social Determinants of Health: The Solid Facts*, 2nd edn. Copenhagen: WHO.

5 Resilience and change: the relationship of work to health

Mel Bartley and Jenny Head

Work is no longer taken for granted, either in the lives of individuals or in the discourse on health and health inequality. Beginning in the 1980s, the classical literature on work hazards began to be supplemented and changed by four major new topics of interest. The first of these was prompted by the widespread economic crises experienced in Organization for Economic Cooperation and Development (OECD) nations. The second was the increasing evidence that the psychosocial conditions of work, not just physical hazards, might play a role in explaining population health patterns. The third and most recent has arisen from the increasing participation of women in the labour force unmatched by a commensurate rise in men's participation in domestic labour. Finally, social policy commentators have increasingly highlighted rising rates of economic inactivity in men (see Chapter 15 for an overview of the changing nature of work).

There are two aspects to the decrease in levels of economic activity; an increasingly feminized labour force is becoming truncated at both ends of the age range. It now takes longer for a young person to establish a work career and it is less likely that workers over the age of 50 will remain economically active than was the case in the 1950s, 1960s and 1970s. But even in the prime working age range, rates of non-participation in work among men have risen dramatically, in large part due to increasing psychological work disability (Henderson *et al.* 2005)

Work as curse and blessing

Attempts to link disease to industrial conditions have always been fraught with difficulty (Blane *et al.* 1998; Evans and Kantrowitz 2002). Moreover it has been argued that the long-term neglect of physical work hazards has been at the expense of the ability of social epidemiology to understand fully the environmental and occupational causes of health inequality (Blane *et al.* 1998; Evans and Kantrowitz 2002).

Despite its hazards, work is highly valued by individuals, and is considered in sociological terms as a central social role (Siegrist 2000). In industrialized nations, employment in an organization of some kind is the major source of income for the greater part of the population. But over and above monetary reward, work is seen to provide essential parts of the individual's sense of identity (Warr 1983, 1987). Research on unemployment and health in the 1980s and 1990s showed that mortality risk was increased in the un-employed, even in nations where generous welfare policies replaced a high proportion of the income of the unemployed (Iversen *et al.* 1987; Moser *et al.* 1987; Bartley 1994).

Although very little researched, it is clear that workers in heavy industry operated with a clear calculus of risk and reward in mind. Heavy and dirty work was worthwhile in so far as it conferred a reasonable living standard and a sense of self worth. In fact, in some industries it was precisely the danger of the work that formed an important part of the self concept of those who experienced it (Hayes 2002; Zoller 2003). Not only did the sense of danger create feelings of solidarity, mutual respect and support among the workers themselves, but their families and communities also shared this.

Work and alienation

At the height of the rapid and dangerous process of industrialization in the nineteenth century, Marx and Engels made the distinction between the human potential of work and work as alienated labour (Sayers 1988). Viewing purposeful activity as self realization, they condemned industrial conditions at the time for destroying the minds and bodies of workers instead of helping to realize their potential. Thus the double-sided nature of work, as both a source of danger, exhaustion, routine boredom and restriction of life on the one hand, and as a source of identity, self realization and life satisfaction on the other, has a long history.

In the current epidemiological debates on the causes of health inequality considered below, there is a tendency to oppose materialist theories, which see health inequality as a product largely of physical hazards of work and poverty, against psychosocial theory which places more emphasis on the experience of work stress, low autonomy and lack of control and social support at work (for further consideration of stress, autonomy, social support and welfare, see Chapters 4 and 6). For Marx and Engels the private ownership of the means of production meant that the factory or business owner had both the power to impose alienated working conditions and to withdraw the ability to work altogether.

A further aspect of health and wellbeing is the nature of relationships at work. It is now known that the emotional and practical support that can be exchanged by co-workers can be an important defence of psychological health (Johnson and Hall 1988; Hibbard and Pope 1992; Johnson *et al.* 1996; Stansfeld *et al.* 1997a, 1997b), to the extent that the loss of a job endangers mental health more or less regardless of the financial consequences of unemployment (Bartley 1994).

Changing patterns of work and the consequences for health

Perhaps the most important strand of literature on work and health now focuses on the radical changes that have effected the labour force since the early 1980s, in the UK and the USA first of all, but then increasingly in all industrial nations (Martin and Rowthorn 1986; Nickell and Quintini 2002). These changes can be characterized as the decline of the heavy industries that gave rise to the prosperity of high-income countries such as the USA, Japan and those in Europe. Many of the processes involved could be automated, which reduced the need for workers. Other processes could be outsourced to low- and middle-income countries where wages are lower.

These trends effected the workforces of the high-income industrial nations, in many ways detrimentally. The heavy industries in the early and mid twentieth century had required a mass labour force of skilled, semi skilled and unskilled workers. The more elaborate skills needed were largely conferred in the course of apprenticeships offered by individual companies, often in partnership with trades unions. Entry into a skilled trade required serving time as an apprentice. The apprenticeship system, though open to abuses, resulted in a form of socialization, fostering collective identity and a sense of common interests as well as skill development (Rhodes 1994; Mortimer and Larson 2002).

A succession of legislative changes in the 1970s and 1980s weakened the ability of trades unions to defend or improve pay levels, in particular by secondary action in which union members picketed workplaces other than their own. The sharp decline in relative pay levels of manual workers that occurred during this period needs to be seen in this light, as well as in the context of changes in industrial structure (Nickell and Quintini 2002).

Figure 5.1 shows the way in which the occupational composition of the labour force of Great Britain changed over the 30 year period from 1971. At the beginning of this period, managers, professionals and higher-level administrators made up around a quarter of the workforce, while skilled craft workers and semi skilled plant and machine operatives accounted for 35 per cent. By 2000, fully 41 per cent of the labour force consisted of managers and professionals, while the share of craft workers and machine operatives had shrunk to 20 per cent.

Figure 5.2 shows change in the types of industry people worked in over the period from 1978 to 2005. The numbers employed in manufacturing declined by around 50 per cent, from around 7 million to just over 3 million, while the numbers of jobs in banking and finance surged from under 3 million to over 6 million. It should be noticed that these figures refer to numbers of jobs, and the number of jobs in the economy overall had grown during the period. But, taken together, Figures 5.1 and 5.2 give some impression of the scale of the changes in what has constituted a typical job during the last 30 years or so. It will also be evident that many of the jobs that have been lost are ones that carry a heavier burden of physical hazard.

Table 5.1 shows the rate of fatal injuries and non fatal injuries that necessitated three or more days' absence from work for employees according to their type of occupation in 2004–5. In addition, 1974 saw within the UK the introduction of the Health and Safety at Work Act, legislation aimed at lowering the number of job related injuries and deaths. Since that year, the rate of fatal injuries to employees has fallen by 76 per cent, from 2.9 per 100,000 employees to 0.7, and non-fatal injuries by a similar amount. Of this reduction, the Health and Safety Executive (HSE) has attributed 24 per cent of the reduction in deaths and 50 per cent of the reduction in injuries to changes in the nature of employment. It is possible that these changes in both the nature of work and in health and safety enforcement may be one reason for the rapid increase in life expectancy, especially life expectancy of those in late working age, that has taken place since the mid 1970s (Anonymous 2003; Shaw 2004). This has yet to be thoroughly investigated.

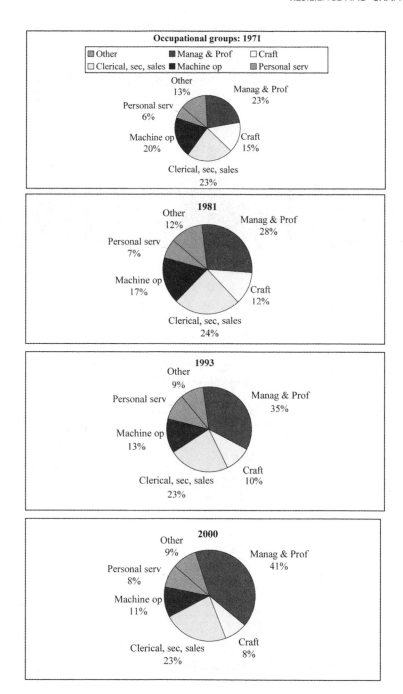

Figure 5.1 Change in occupational composition of the labour force 1971–2000
Source: Drever (1995)

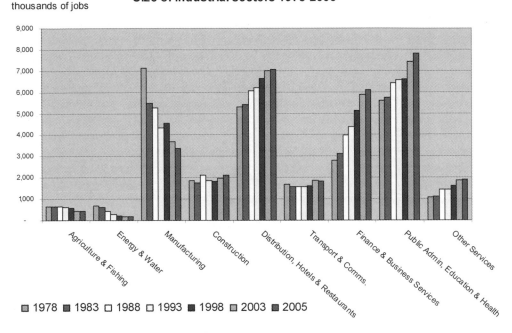

Figure 5.2 Change in sizes of industrial sectors 1978–2005
Source: http://www.statistics.gov.uk/statbase/product.asp?vlnk=8286

Table 5.1 Work injury rates in different occupational groups, 2004–5

	Injuries: rate per 100,000 employees	
Occupational group	*Fatal injuries*	*Non-fatal injuries needing 3+ days away from work*
Managers and senior officials	0.3	89.2
Professional	0.1	138.4
Associate professional and technical	0.3	335.3
Administrative and secretarial	–	80.6
Skilled trades	1.6	746.1
Personal service	0.1	516.0
Sales	–	316.8
Process, plant and machine operatives	3.0	1733.7
Elementary occupations	1.2	943.8

Stress: the new industrial hazard?

The major exception to this benign trend in work-related ill health has been in the occurrence of illnesses due to stress, which increased between 1974 and 2004/5 from 820 to 1500 per 100,000 employees. In other words, stress-related illness has almost doubled over the period (HSE statistics website www.hse.gov.uk/statistics/history/index.htm).

Research on work stress has a complex history, and is at present an area of some controversy. Confusion can easily arise over a number of related issues. The definition and measurement of stress has varied over time, and different operational definitions give different relationships to other aspects of employment conditions (Macleod *et al.* 2002; Macleod and Davey Smith 2003; Eaker *et al.* 2004). Some of the most important research on work stress and health is that based on a measure initially developed by Robert Karasek, who focused on the combination of work demands and control. Karasek's early studies seemed to show that employees whose jobs combined high demands and low control, a combination he termed job strain, were at higher risk of ill health, in particular heart disease (Karasek *et al.* 1981, 1988; Pieper *et al.* 1985; Reed *et al.* 1989; Schnall *et al.* 1990; Karasek 1996). However, other studies in different populations have not all borne out these findings. For example, high work demand tends to be reported more frequently by those in professional and senior managerial positions than those in less powerful types of white-collar jobs. Because of the strong relationship between the general social status of an occupation and health, high work demand in some studies is actually related to better rather than poorer health (Macleod *et al.* 2002). If asked directly whether they experience stress at work, those who answer positively are not usually found to be in worse health than those who report low stress (Macleod *et al.* 2005).

However, questions on the degree of control and autonomy at work, or on the balance between effort and reward, have also been widely used in health research, and more often than not found to yield more confirmatory evidence of a relationship between these forms of work stress and poorer health (for further discussion of autonomy, see Chapters 4 and 6). Even where studies take account of the fact that some people may tend to report both poor health and low control or rewards at work because of depressed mood, these relationships are still strongly present (Bosma *et al.* 1998; Stansfeld *et al.* 1998a). When investigating health in mixed populations of both white- and blue-collar workers, some studies have also found risks of coronary disease to be higher where high demands are coupled with low control (Hallqvist *et al.* 1998; Kuper and Marmot 2003), or with low perceived rewards in terms of pay and status (Siegrist 1996; Kivimäki *et al.* 2002; Kuper *et al.* 2002). Even higher risk of cardiovascular ill health has been found in those who combine imbalances in both work demands and control and efforts versus rewards (de Jonge *et al.* 2000; Peter *et al.* 2002).

Despite the controversy, this literature has given rise to a demand from government agencies such as the UK HSE for a greater understanding of the role that may be played by management practices in producing different forms of work stress, an understanding that would lead to improvements in practices and thereby in health.

Research had also shown that social support at work, from co-workers or supervisors, could protect against stress factors (Johnson *et al.* 1996; Roy *et al.* 1998; Steptoe 2000). A new concept of isostrain has arisen, which refers to the combination of high work strain combined with low social support, and which seems to be more strongly related to some health outcomes than either factor on its own (Chandola *et al.* 2006).

Work as a source of resilience

Some time ago, however, Steptoe, one of the leading psycho-physiological researchers in this area, and his colleagues appealed for a consideration of the role of personal resilience to make full sense of what is sometimes a confusing and contradictory mass of research findings (Steptoe 1991; Steptoe *et al.* 2005). This research construct of resilience appears to be seen as a personal characteristic, derived either from inherited constitution or from early life experiences, or both of these. There does seem to be a large degree of variability between persons in the reactions to the kinds of stressors measured conventionally in studies of work and health.

While drawing attention to resilience in the face of work stress has been an important innovation for research in this area, recent writing on resilience has tended more towards conceptualizing it as a product of environment as much as deriving from the individual. Such a view echoes Marx and Engels' concept of work as a source of meaning, and potential source of resilience. Stressors become seen not only as hazardous exposures but also, potentially, as factors that strengthen the individual both psychologically and physically. For one thing, this conceptualization immediately makes sense of the paradox that appears to be produced by high-status white-collar workers reporting more job demands, higher levels of stress and at the same time having reduced risk of many forms of ill health (Macleod *et al.* 2005). For these workers the perception that much is demanded of them and that they carry a weight of responsibility is a source of pride and wellbeing. High perceived demands are therefore not linked to ill health when they are accompanied by rewards in the form of high pay and status within the organization.

An example of the way in which higher pay and status may be able to protect the health of workers can be taken from the Whitehall II Study. This study has followed some 10,000 male and female London-based civil servants from ages 35–55 in the mid-1980s to the present day. The study includes a large number of measures of physical and mental health. Among these is a measure of attachment style, which is an indicator of how easy or difficult an individual finds everyday relationships to others, at work or at home (Bifulco 2002). Many previous studies have shown that an insecure, anxious or avoidant attachment style is related to higher levels of depression and anxiety (Shaver and Mikulincer 2002; Scharf *et al.* 2004). Figure 5.3 shows the way in which occupational grade in the Civil Service appears to have protected study members with the less secure attachment styles from depression. Those with the less secure attachment styles had higher scores on a depression scale derived from the General Health Questionnaire, regardless of their grade of employment. But the interesting thing is that this difference is so much greater in the lower (Grade 3) than in the higher (Grade 1) grades of employment. The degree to which the relationship between attachment and depression differed according to grade was significant (p<0.05).

Work as a source of resilience in women

The Whitehall II data shown here only include men, because in the 1980s when the study began there were so few women in the top grades of the Civil Service that a reliable

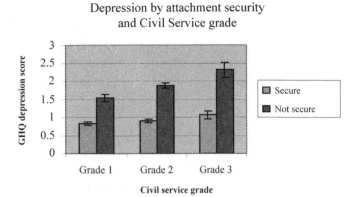

Figure 5.3 Is work a source of resilience in mental health?

comparison could not be made. However, there is further evidence on the ways in which work contributes to wellbeing in women. Ever since the proportion of women in the labour force of the USA and UK began to rise, health researchers have inquired into the impact of multiple roles. At first, it was suspected that adding the burdens of paid employment to those of care for the home and family would endanger women's health (Verbrugge 1983; Repetti *et al.* 1989; Martikainen 1995). However, the vast majority of research in this area repeatedly finds that women who are paid employees as well as spouses and mothers have the best health, according to a variety of different health indicators (La Rosa 1988; Weatherall *et al.* 1994; Steptoe *et al.* 2000). A few studies have considered the importance of work quality, defined in a variety of ways, and reported that paid work that is perceived to be of high quality is more protective to health than less rewarding employment (Bullers 1994). In some American studies of cardiovascular disease, women in manual occupations were found to have greatly increased risk, and there were indications that low levels of workplace social support may have been one factor (Hall *et al.* 1993).

Apart from the Whitehall II study (Rael *et al.* 1995; Stansfeld *et al.* 1997b, 1998b), not a great deal of research seems to have been done on the relationship to women's health of social support at work (Repetti *et al.* 1989). The best example is perhaps a qualitative study by Hochschild, which vividly depicts the contrast between the social and emotional situations at work and home of many women workers (Hochschild 1997). Hochschild highlights two issues in particular: differential social support is one, but differential power is another. Among the women with managerial jobs, the ability to command others is a major attraction of the workplace over the home. Among the assembly workers, the fellowship and support of colleagues is contrasted, very starkly in some cases, with the constant demands of children and in some cases abusive behaviour of husbands. The beneficial effect on health of occupying the role of worker as well as that of wife and mother has also been found to be associated with social support from work colleagues in some large-scale studies (Hibbard and Pope 1992).

The relationship of work to health can be seen to be complex and multifaceted. Recent research seems to indicate with increasing strength that work is a high positive aspect of life for the great majority of people. There is also, however, a great deal of unrealized potential in modern economies. At the same time as work has become less physically arduous and dangerous, and often more creative, labour markets have also tended to become more flexible and fragmented, with lower levels of job security and a more difficult passage from adolescence to a stable work career.

These changes have made some of the positive aspects of work more visible even as they begin to disappear. Even relatively low-skilled routine work was often a refuge for troubled young people, offering them stable relationships with others as they developed their adult identities. However, these work roles could then act as a trap, and as a disincentive to further self-development. In the contemporary labour market, working lives, particularly for many women, will be more dynamic and fulfilling than would have seemed possible for their parents. However, social policy has not yet discovered an alternative way to provide a secure base from which all workers may be enabled to make full use of their talents and energies.

References

Anonymous (2003) Annual mortality report: life expectancy increase, *Public Health Reports*, 118: 275–6.

Bartley, M. (1994) Unemployment and ill health: understanding the relationship, *Journal of Epidemiology and Community Health*, 48: 333–7.

Bifulco, A. (2002) Attachment style measurement: a clinical and epidemiological perspective, *Attachment and Human Development*, 4: 180–8.

Blane, D., Bartley, M. and Smith, G.D. (1998) Disease aetiology and materialist explanations of socioeconomic mortality differentials: a research note, *European Journal of Public Health*, 8: 259–60.

Bosma, H., Peter, R., Siegrist, J. and Marmot, M. (1998) Two alternative job stress models and the risk of coronary heart disease, *American Journal of Public Health*, 88: 68–74.

Bullers, S. (1994) Women's roles and health: the mediating effect of perceived control, *Women and Health*, 22: 11–30.

Chandola, T., Brunner, E. and Marmot, M. (2006) Chronic stress and work and the metabolic syndrome: prospective study, *British Medical Journal*, 332: 521–5.

de Jonge, J., Bosma, H., Peter, R. and Siegrist, J. (2000) Job strain, effort–reward imbalance and employee wellbeing: a large-scale cross-sectional study, *Social Science and Medicine*, 50: 1317–27.

Drever, P. (1995) *Occupational Health*. London: HMSO.

Eaker, E.D., Sullivan, L.M., Kelly-Hayes, M., D'Agostino Sr, R. and Benjamin, E. (2004) Does job strain increase the risk for coronary heart disease or death in men and women? The Framingham offspring study, *American Journal of Epidemiology*, 159.

Evans, G.W. and Kantrowitz, E. (2002) Socioeconomic status and health: the potential role of environmental risk exposure, *Annual Review of Public Health*, 23: 303–31.

Hall, E.M., Johnson, J.V. and Tsou, T.S. (1993) Women, occupation, and risk of cardiovascular morbidity and mortality, *Occupational Medicine*, 8: 709–19.

Hallqvist, J., Diderichsen, F., Theorell, T., Reuterwall, C. and Ahlbom, A. (1998) Is the effect of job strain on myocardial infarction risk due to interaction between high psychological demands and low decision latitude? Results from Stockholm Heart Epidemiology Program (SHEEP), *Social Science and Medicine*, 46: 1405–15.

Hayes, N. (2002) Did manual workers want industrial welfare? Canteens, latrines and masculinity on British building sites 1918–1970, *Journal of Social History*, 35: 637–58.

Henderson, M., Glozier, N. and Holland Elliott, K. (2005) Long term sickness absence is caused by common conditions and needs managing, *British Medical Journal*, 330: 802–3.

Hibbard, J.H. and Pope, C.R. (1992) Women's employment, social support, and mortality, *Women and Health*, 18: 119–33.

Hochschild, A.R. (1997) *The Time Bind: When Work Becomes Home and Home Becomes Work.* New York: Metropolitan Books.

Iversen, L., Andersen, O., Andersen, P.K., Christoffersen, K. and Keiding, N. (1987) Unemployment and mortality in Denmark, *British Medical Journal*, 295: 879–84.

Johnson, J.V. and Hall, E.M. (1988) Job strain, work place social support, and cardiovascular disease: a cross-sectional study of a random sample of the Swedish working population, *American Journal of Public Health*, 78: 1336–42.

Johnson, J.V., Stewart, W., Hall, E.M., Fredlund, P. and Theorell, T. (1996) Long-term psychosocial work-environment and cardiovascular mortality among Swedish men, *American Journal of Public Health*, 86: 324–31.

Karasek, R. (1996) Job strain and the prevalence and outcome of coronary-artery disease, *Circulation*, 94: 1140–1.

Karasek, R., Baker, D., Marxer, F., Ahlbom, A. and Theorell, T. (1981) Job decision latitude, job demands, and cardiovascular-disease – a prospective-study of Swedish men, *American Journal of Public Health*, 71. 694–705.

Karasek, R.A., Theorell, T., Schwartz, J.E., Schnall, P.L., Pieper, C.F. and Michela, J.L. (1988) Job characteristics in relation to the prevalence of myocardial infarction in the United States Health Examination Survey (HES) and the Health and Nutrition Examination Survey (HANES), *American Journal of Public Health*, 78: 910–18.

Kivimäki, M., Leino-Arjas, P., Luukkonen, R., Riihimäki, H., Vahtera, J. and Kirjonen, J. (2002) Work stress and risk of cardiovascular mortality: prospective cohort study of industrial employees, *British Medical Journal*, 325: 857.

Kuper, H. and Marmot, M. (2003) Job strain, job demands, decision latitude, and risk of coronary heart disease within the Whitehall II study, *Journal of Epidemiology and Community Health*, 57: 147–53.

Kuper, H., Singh Manoux, A., Siegrist, J. and Marmot, M. (2002) When reciprocity fails: effort–reward imbalance in relation to coronary heart disease and health functioning within the Whitehall II study, *Occupational and Environmental Medicine*, 59: 777–84.

La Rosa, J.H. (1988) Women, work, and health: employment as a risk factor for coronary heart disease, *American Journal of Obstetrics and Gynecology*, 158: 1597–602.

Macleod, J. and Davey Smith, G. (2003) Psychosocial factors and public health: a suitable case for treatment? *Journal of Epidemiology and Community Health*, 89: 565–70.

Macleod, J., Davey Smith, G., Heslop, P., Metcalfe, C., Carroll, D. and Hart, C. (2002) Psychological stress and cardiovascular disease: empirical demonstration of bias in a prospective observational study of Scottish men, *British Medical Journal*, 56: 1247–51.

Macleod, J., Davey Smith, G., Metcalfe, C. and Hart, C. (2005) Is subjective social status a more important determinant of health than objective social status? Evidence from a prospective observational study of Scottish men. *Social Science and Medicine*, 61: 1916–29.

Martikainen, P. (1995) Women's employment, marriage, motherhood and mortality: a test of the multiple role and role accumulation hypotheses, *Social Science and Medicine*, 40: 199–212.

Martin, R. and Rowthorn, R. (1986) *The Geography of De-industrialisation*. Basingstoke: Macmillan.

Mortimer, J.T. and Larson, R.W. (eds) (2002) *The Changing Adolescent Experience*. Cambridge: Cambridge University Press.

Moser, K.A., Goldblatt, P.O., Fox, A.J. and Jones, D.R. (1987) Unemployment and mortality – comparison of the 1971 and 1981 longitudinal-study census samples, *British Medical Journal*, 294: 86–90.

Nickell, S. and Quintini, G. (2002) The recent performance of the UK labour market, *Oxford Review of Economic Policy*, 18(2): 202–20.

Peter, R., Siegrist, J., Hallqvist, J., Reuterwall, C. and Theorell, T. (2002) Psychosocial work environment and myocardial infarction: improving risk estimation by combining two complementary job stress models in the SHEEP Study, *Journal of Epidemiology and Community Health*, 56: 294–300.

Pieper, C., Karasek, R. and Schwartz, J. (1985) The relationship of job dimensions to coronary heart-disease risk-factors, *American Journal of Epidemiology*, 122: 540–1.

Rael, E.G., Stansfeld, S.A., Shipley, M., Head, J., Feeney, A. and Marmot, M. (1995) Sickness absence in the Whitehall II study, London: the role of social support and material problems, *Journal of Epidemiology and Community Health*, 49: 474–81.

Reed, D.M., Lacroix, A.Z., Karasek, R.A., Miller, D. and Maclean, C.A. (1989) Occupational strain and the incidence of coronary heart-disease, *American Journal of Epidemiology*, 129: 495–502.

Repetti, R.L., Matthews, K.A. and Waldron, I. (1989) Employment and women's health: effects of paid employment on women's mental and physical health, *American Psychologist*, 44: 1394–401.

Rhodes, J.E. (1994) Older and wiser: mentoring relationship in childhood and adolescence, *Journal of Primary Prevention*, 14: 187–96.

Roy, M.P., Steptoe, A. and Kirschbaum, C. (1998) Life events and social support as moderators of individual differences in cardiovascular and cortisol reactivity, *Journal of Personality and Social Psychology*, 75: 1273–81.

Sayers, S. (1988) The need to work, in R.E. Pahl (ed.) *On Work*. Oxford: Basil Blackwell.

Scharf, M., Mayseless, O. and Kivenson-Baron, I. (2004) Adolescents' attachment representations and developmental tasks in emerging adulthood, *Developmental Psychology*, 40: 430–44.

Schnall, P.L., Pieper, C., Schwartz, J.E., Karasek, R.A., Schlussel, Y. and Devereux, C. (1990) The relationship between job strain, workplace diastolic blood pressure, and left-ventricular mass index – results of a case-control study, *Journal of the American Medical Association*, 263: 1929–35.

Shaver, P.R. and Mikulincer, M. (2002) Attachment-related psychodynamics, *Attachment and Human Development*, 4: 133–61.

Shaw, C. (2004) Interim 2003-based national population projections for the United Kingdom and constituent countries, *Population Trends*, 118: 6–16.

Siegrist, J. (1996) Adverse health effects of high-effort/low-reward conditions, *Journal of Occupational Health Psychology*, 1: 27–41.

Siegrist, J. (2000) Place, social exchange and health: proposed sociological framework, *Social Science and Medicine*, 51: 1283–93.

Stansfeld, S.A., Fuhrer, R., Head, J., Ferrie, J. and Shipley, M. (1997a) Work and psychiatric disorder in the Whitehall II Study, *Journal of Psychosomatic Research*, 43: 73–81.

Stansfeld, S.A., Rael, E.G., Head, J., Shipley, M. and Marmot, M. (1997b) Social support and psychiatric sickness absence: a prospective study of British civil servants, *Psychologie Medicale*, 27: 35–48.

Stansfeld, S.A., Bosma, H., Hemingway, H. and Marmot, M.G. (1998a) Psychosocial work characteristics and social support as predictors of SF-36 health functioning: the Whitehall II study, *Psychosomatic Medicine*, 60: 247–55.

Stansfeld, S.A., Fuhrer, R. and Shipley, M.J. (1998b) Types of social support as predictors of psychiatric morbidity in a cohort of British civil servants (Whitehall II Study), *Psychologie Medicale*, 28: 881–92.

Steptoe, A. (1991) Invited review: the links between stress and illness, *Journal of Psychosomatic Research*, 35: 633–44.

Steptoe, A. (2000) Stress, social support and cardiovascular activity over the working day, *International Journal of Psychophysiology*, 37: 299–308.

Steptoe, A., Lundwall, K. and Cropley, M. (2000) Gender, family structure and cardiovascular activity during the working day and evening, *Social Science and Medicine*, 50: 531–9.

Steptoe, A., Wardle, J. and Marmot, M. (2005) Positive affect and health-related neuroendocrine, cardiovascular, and inflammatory processes, *Proceedings of the National Academy of Sciences of the United States of America*, 102: 6508–12.

Verbrugge, L.M. (1983) Multiple roles and physical health of women and men, *Journal of Health and Social Behavior*, 24: 16–30.

Warr, P. (1983) Work, jobs and unemployment, *Bulletin of the British Psychological Society*, 36: 305–11.

Warr, P. (1987) *Work, Unemployment and Mental Health*. London: Oxford University Press.

Weatherall, R., Joshi, H. and Macran, S. (1994) Double burden or double blessing? Employment, motherhood and mortality in the Longitudinal Study of England and Wales, *Social Science and Medicine*, 38: 285–97.

Zoller, H.M. (2003) Health on the line: identity and disciplinary control in employee occupational health and safety discourse, *Journal of Applied Comunication Research*, 31: 118–39.

6 Social capital, social exclusion and wellbeing

Yaojun Li

The concept of social capital is both seductive and infuriating. It is seductive because it has captivated the imagination of lay people, policy makers and academics alike. Discussions on this topic recur in popular media, government documents and academic journals from a wide range of social science disciplines (see Keane 1998; Field 2003; Edwards 2004 for good overviews). Since the mid 1990s the number of publications on this topic has increased exponentially so that now there are around 300 to 400 publications in the English language alone each year. Yet, the concept of social capital is also infuriating, defying characterization, measurement or falsification in any simple, straightforward and precise manner. Unlike human capital, economic capital, physical capital or even cultural capital, where both proponents and opponents have some clear idea of and consensus about what the terms refer to, social capital as a concept is elusive, nebulous and does not easily yield to empirical, especially quantitative, investigation. Critics, unsurprisingly, find the concept chaotic and ambiguous (Fine 2001: 155; see also Skocpol 1996; Kadushin 2004). Here the focus of analysis will be on the theoretical rigour of seminal versions of the theory, with special attention being given to implications for operational feasibility in quantitative analysis.

Writers usually seen as pioneers in social capital research (Bourdieu 1984, 1986; Coleman 1988; Putnam 2000; Lin 2001) identify social capital as a human resource residing in social networks. Their differences lie in the emphasis given to the instrumental, individual value of social capital on the one hand, and its contribution to bolstering a communal, civic spirit on the other. On an imaginary line of a continuum, with instrumental value on the left and civic spirit on the right, Lin and Bourdieu might place themselves on the left, Coleman centre left and Putnam on the right. Lin's interest in social capital is primarily concerned with explaining occupational attainment (Lin *et al.* 1981; Lin 1999a, 1999b, 2001) although he also uses the concept to explain depression (Lin *et al.* 1999). His basic assumption is that the resources an individual can access and utilize depend on the extent of social ties, the position of the contact and the strength of tie with the contact. This thesis can be called the strength of strong ties, which complements that of the strength of weak ties developed by Granovetter (1973, 1974, 1985; see also Burt 1992, 2000 for a more recent application). Lin's own research and that of many others in this tradition have demonstrated the research value of this approach in accounting for occupational attainment although survey instruments using this approach are not fully available in the UK.

In contrast to the operational value of what Coleman (1988) calls the methodological individualism found in Lin's work, Bourdieu's notion of social capital is conceptually inspiring but difficult to use. For him, social capital is the sum of resources, actual or virtual, that accrue to individuals or groups through their networks of institutionalized relationships (Bourdieu and Wacquant 1992: 119). Bourdieu's theoretical work has been highly influential in European research as it allows social capital, cultural capital and economic capital to be investigated together so that insight can be gained into the intergenerational transmission of class advantages. In this sense, social capital is seen as a dimension of social exclusion such that the networks between people also involve non-ties with outsiders who are excluded from social capital (Li et al. 2003). For him it is a residual category to explain how elites can use networks for instrumental gains when they do not have sufficient cultural or economic capital. The crucial thing, for Bourdieu, is that if cultural capital and economic capital function properly, there is no need for social capital since highly educated parents can instil in their children the *habitus* for educational attainment and well-resourced parents can buy a good education to ensure occupational success (Bourdieu 1986). For present purposes, it suffices to note that while Bourdieu's theory of social capital offers insight in stratification research, it lacks the operational feasibility for large-scale survey research.

Space limitations do not allow for an analysis of Coleman's theory, except to note that his functionalist approach has been heavily criticized as being tautological (Lin 2001) and his empirical work for being flawed (Field 2003). It is Robert Putnam (1993, 2000) who has generated the most heated debate and made social capital a priority in research within social science disciplines. For him, social capital refers to connections between people; social networks and the norms of reciprocity and trustworthiness that arise from them (2000: 19). This definition is a conceptual riddle and has been a source of much of the controversy since it combines both connections, as causes, and norms of reciprocity and trust, as consequences. Yet by focusing on the causal element it is possible to draw attention to something quite often neglected in the current debate.

In his earlier work, Putnam (1993) saw civic participation as the main source of social capital since the experience of engagement in civic associations enables people to learn how to reconcile differences and to work cooperatively together. Yet, in his later work, Putnam realized the importance of, and accordingly placed greater emphasis upon, informal networks such as friendship (Putnam 2000: 95). This distinction between formal and informal social connections, with the latter as the greater source of social capital, is not yet fully appreciated but it is the starting point of the present research.

Measuring social capital, wellbeing and socioeconomic factors

For proponents of the concept, social capital resides in social networks, whether formal or informal. Although Putnam's work does not make methodological advances with regard to social capital measurement, it is conceptually vigorous enough to inspire others. The work described in this chapter draws on Putnam to develop social capital measures (Li et al. 2005) using data from the British Household Panel Survey (BHPS). The BHPS began in

1991 and samples around 5000 households and 10,000 individuals each year. Although some of the original sample members left the survey, new members are added each year, and the sample remains appropriately representative of the population as a whole in each wave (Taylor *et al.* 2002).

The social capital questions, available in Waves 7 and 8 of the survey, can be conceptualized as falling into three types or dimensions. Details on constructing the latent scores for the three dimensions of social capital are published elsewhere (Li *et al.* 2005). Here is a brief summary.

Neighbourhood attachment refers to the degree to which people feel that they belong to the neighbourhood, cherish the friendships cultivated with neighbours and perceive that having good neighbours can give them practical value, like being able to obtain advice and borrow things, or to have frequent chats with. All these are important aspects of informal social capital.

Social network measures the strength of ties with people beyond immediate family: with friends who may, or may not, be living in the same neighbourhood. It asks whether people have friends whose support they can rely on for practical and emotional problems. Many people may not know the names of their neighbours but may call on friends for help who are located hundreds of miles away.

Civic participation is usually calculated in studies on social capital by using civic membership as an indicator of social capital (Hall 1999; Paxton 1999; Putnam 2000; Li *et al.* 2003, 2006). Most studies use descriptive methods by counting the number of such memberships. The measure developed here calculates the level of civic involvement as obtained from the underlying scores in the voluntary associations. The level of civic participation thus obtained is a reasonable measure of formal social capital emanating from involvement in voluntary associations.

A unique feature of the BHPS is that its longitudinal nature allows assessment of the effects of explanatory variables upon outcomes of interest measured at a later time. According to Helliwell and Putnam (2004: 1437) this research design is necessary if the causal effects of social capital on wellbeing are to be explored. As the social capital data are drawn from Waves 7 and 8, wellbeing variables from Wave 9 are used: general state of health, psychological distress and overall satisfaction with life. All three measures are widely used in social research in the UK and other countries (for health, see Ross and Wu 1995; Hertzman *et al.* 2001; Chandola *et al.* 2003; Pevalin and Rose 2003).

The framework for analysis is shown in Figure 6.1. The research design adopted here has some advantages. First, the analysis of dependent and independent variables measured at different time points will help avoid the kind of reverse causality whereby people who are healthier, happier and more satisfied with life are more likely to participate in formal and informal networks. Second, the inclusion of health status as a covariate in modelling happiness and satisfaction helps remove the confounding effect that the observed positive correlation between social capital and happiness may be both due to health. In other words, healthier people are more likely both to engage in social networking and to report greater happiness or satisfaction, but the association would disappear once health status is taken into account.

As for outcome variables, the health and life satisfaction measures are self-explanatory. With regard to the happiness measure, the Likert scale of the General Health Questionnaire (GHQ12) was adopted. This is a summary measure of the 12 items in the

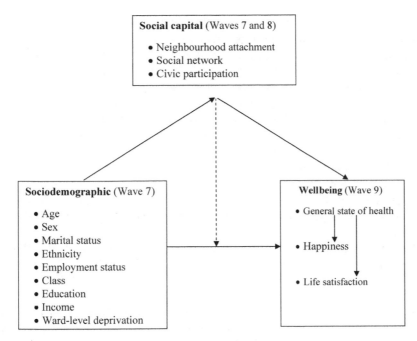

Figure 6.1 Sociodemographic factors, social capital and wellbeing indicators

Notes:

1 Data on sociodemographic factors are drawn from Wave 7 (1997), those on social capital from Waves 7 and 8, and those on wellbeing from Wave 9 of the BHPS.

2 Solid lines denote direct effects and dotted lines denote mediator effects. Thus we assume that health status is both determined by sociodemographic and social capital factors, and has an impact on happiness and life satisfaction.

GHQ and is coded with a minimum of 0 for least depressed and a maximum of 36 for most depressed. The measure has been validated (Argyle 1989; Pevalin 2000) and is widely used by medical researchers and psychiatrists as an indicator of strain or psychological distress (Gardner and Oswald 2006: 322). It is noted here that, as higher scores in the satisfaction variable denote greater satisfaction with life, for the sake of consistency in the interpretation of results the scores have been reversed so that higher values denote less depression or greater happiness. Hereafter it is called the happiness variable. The analysis of both happiness and life satisfaction data is necessary for exploring the relative effects of social capital. This is because self-ratings of happiness tend to reflect short-term, situation-dependent expressions of mood in contrast to the more stable evaluations evoked by life satisfaction questions (Helliwell and Putnam 2004: 1435). The analysis here will allow an assessment of whether life satisfaction is indeed a longer-term evaluation than happiness.

It is important to say a few words on the control variables. Apart from the social capital measures, an assessment is made of the effects of sociodemographic attributes that are often found to influence wellbeing. These include age, sex, marital status, ethnicity, employment status, class, education, income and local social deprivation (see Carstairs and Morris 1989; Buck 2000). Blanchflower and Oswald (2004), for example, show that wellbeing is U-shaped in age, that a lasting marriage is worth more than widowhood, and that money buys happiness. Wilkinson (2002) argues that having a job brings not only material rewards but, much more importantly, the esteem and self-respect crucial for wellbeing. Unemployment can trigger depression, doubt of self-worth, diffidence, isolation and loss of social contact that will lead to distress and induce a whole range of psychological and physiological problems (for further discussion of employment, unemployment and health see Chapters 4, 5 and 15).

Ethnicity is rarely found in social capital and wellbeing research in Britain as most ethnic research has focused on racial discrimination in occupational and educational attainment (Karn 1997; Modood and Berthoud 1997; White 2002). Lin (1999b) suggests that, apart from socioeconomic disadvantages, ethnic groups might have different sentiments, which may prevent minority groups from forming network ties with the majority groups. The effect of ethnicity on social capital and wellbeing is investigated here (for background discussion to the epidemiology of ethnicity in Britain, see Chapter 7).

Although existing research has shown profound and persisting class differences in social capital generation in the UK (Hall 1999; Li *et al.* 2003, 2005, 2006), relatively little class analysis has been conducted on wellbeing, and it is not clear whether class has any explanatory power in this regard. A three way class schema is utilized here (Goldthorpe *et al.* 1987). It distinguishes the service class, the intermediate class and the manual working class. Like most research in this area, the effects of education are assessed. Three levels are differentiated: tertiary, secondary and primary or no qualification.

With regard to income, the standardized household mean income is constructed by taking the total household annual income from all sources divided by the equivalence scale. This is the standard practice adopted by government agencies and the research community in the UK (Jenkins 1999; Li *et al.* 2002). Finally, ward-level social deprivation is included in the analysis. The purpose of this is to try to reduce the atomistic fallacies sometimes attributed to the use of individual level data (Schwartz 1994; Kawachi *et al.* 1997).

All sociodemographic and contextual variables are drawn from Wave 7, social capital data from Waves 7 and 8, and wellbeing data from Wave 9. The Stata 9 statistical package is used for the data management and statistical modelling. All analysis is based on weighted data, analytical weights in descriptive analysis and probability weights in statistical modelling. All models are estimated using pseudo likelihood to account for the weights and clustering, with standard errors, confidence intervals and p values based on a robust estimator of the parameter covariance matrices. Owing to the amount of data presented, standard errors and the 95 per cent confidence intervals are not shown in the tables that follow.

Table 6.1 shows the correlation coefficients between the social capital dimensions and happiness and life satisfaction scores. As a categorical variable, it is not appropriate to include health for use in correlation analysis. The three dimensions of social capital, neighbourhood attachment, social network and civic participation are positively but weakly correlated. People with strong informal social capital tend to be happier and more satisfied with life than those with higher scores on civic participation. There is, unsurprisingly, a much stronger association between happiness and satisfaction (0.553) than between any other pairs. The patterns here support, at a general level, the hypothesis that social capital contributes to happiness and life satisfaction, and that

Table 6.1 Correlation between social capital dimensions, subjective wellbeing and overall satisfaction with life

	1	2	3	4	5
1 Neighbourhood attachment	1.000				
2 Social network	0.147***	1.000			
3 Civic participation	0.115***	0.082***	1.000		
4 Happiness	0.078***	0.134***	0.018†	1.000	
5 Satisfaction with life	0.182***	0.164***	0.051***	0.553***	1.000

†p<0.10, *p<0.05, **p<0.01 and ***p<0.001.
Source: BHPS

informal social support tends to be more important to wellbeing than formal civic engagement (Putnam 2000).

Having looked at the association between social capital and wellbeing at the most general level, the association between sociodemographic attributes with happiness and life satisfaction is considered. Table 6.2 presents three main types of data. Firstly, the last column shows the sample size for different socioeconomic groups. Most of the groups have large sizes but some small groups are included for theoretical reasons. For instance, existing research has shown significant differences between people of Indian and of Pakistani/Bangladeshi origins in terms of socioeconomic conditions (Karn 1997; White 2002). Thus Pakistanis and Bangladeshis are listed as a separate category (N = 33). It is noted here that as there are only 12 Chinese in the sample, they have to be combined with the 'Other' group. Secondly, mean scores and standard deviations for happiness and life satisfaction are presented for each of the sociodemographic groups. Thirdly, the statistical significance is shown between each of the other categories in a variable. For instance, the mean score of happiness for men is 25.8 and that for women is 24.3. Men are on the whole happier than women and their difference is significant at the 0.001 level. On the other hand, no statistically significant difference between men and women in life satisfaction was found.

Table 6.2 Mean scores of happiness and satisfaction with life by sociodemographic attributes

	Happiness		Satisfaction		
	Mean	(SD)	Mean	(SD)	N
Sex					
Male	25.761***	(4.951)	5.268	(1.228)	3468
Female	24.341	(5.514)	5.230	(1.327)	4009
Marital status					
Married	24.939**	(5.215)	5.334***	(1.247)	4454
Single	25.608***	(5.211)	5.132	(1.213)	1769
Divorced/separated/widowed	24.356	(5.679)	5.099	(1.465)	1252
Ethnicity					
White	24.994	(5.278)	5.526	(1.275)	7167
Black	25.044	(6.460)	4.847*	(1.412)	68
Indian	24.135	(5.773)	4.952	(1.549)	89
Pakistani/Bangladeshi	25.234	(6.227)	5.077	(1,239)	33
Chinese/other	24.835	(6.327)	4.811†	(1.575)	60

	Happiness		Satisfaction		
	Mean	(SD)	Mean	(SD)	N
Employment status					
Employed	25.322*	(5.078)	5.253***	(1.133)	4281
Non-employed	24.582	(5.467)	5.287***	(1.441)	2963
Unemployed	24.244	(6.846)	4.643	(1.590)	226
Class					
Service class	25.221	(5.257)	5.285	(1.143)	2248
Intermediate	24.880	(5.274)	5.247	(1.313)	2792
Working class	24.964	(5.357)	5.217	(1.362)	2154
Education					
Tertiary	25.262***	(5.259)	5.237	(1.164)	2384
Secondary	25.292***	(5.086)	5.213†	(1.192)	2281
Primary/none	24.504	(5.491)	5.290	(1.440)	2691
Income					
Top quartile	25.342***	(5.181)	5.367***	(1.072)	1913
2nd	25.505***	(4.952)	5.302***	(1.199)	2065
3rd	24.884***	(5.429)	5.221***	(1.342)	1845
Bottom	24.105	(5.613)	5.067	(1.507)	1632
Social deprivation					
Affluent areas	25.217**	(5.033)	5.311***	(1.193)	2412
Middle	24.981	(5.328)	5.263**	(1.280)	3151
Deprived areas (base)	24.728	(5.625)	5.140	(1.388)	1874
Health					
Excellent/very good	26.478***	(4.240)	5.581***	(1.043)	3388
Good	25.148***	(4.768)	5.245***	(1.198)	2510
Fair/poor	21.519	(6.511)	4.520	(1.558)	1578
All	25.000	(5.307)	5.247	(1.282)	7536

†$p<0.10$, *$p<0.05$, **$p<0.01$ and ***$p<0.001$

With regard to happiness, the data in the last row of Table 6.2 show an overall mean score of 25 (and the median is 26, not shown in the table). This is in conformity with that reported in Gardner and Oswald (2006: 323). A closer look shows patterns in support of previous findings (Lin *et al.* 1999; Blanchflower and Oswald 2004; Helliwell and Putnam 2004; Shields and Wheatley Price 2005; Stutzer and Frey 2006). Thus, apart from the gender differences as noted above, it is found, as expected, that there are significant differences between people with different marital and employment statuses, with different educational qualifications, in different economic situations, living in areas of differing social deprivation and with different health conditions. Only in two aspects are exceptions found: there are no significant class and ethnic differences in terms of happiness. It is known that class and ethnicity are powerful predictors of a whole range of socioeconomic outcomes such as family income, and yet it is surprising to find that the much lower incomes of working class respondents or of Pakistani/Bangladeshi groups are not reflected in their happiness evaluations. The evidence here might be taken as a sign of adaptation (Wilson 1967): the working class or the minority ethnic groups may find their jobs rather unpleasant and their purses quite empty, but this does not necessarily make life distressful. On the other hand, the differences between health groups are by far the most pronounced. People who see their health as in an excellent or very good state report a mean happiness score of 26.5, as against 21.5 for those with fair or poor health ratings. No other variables in the table show differences to a similar magnitude.

With regard to life satisfaction, patterns broadly similar to those on happiness are found. Thus, people who were married, employed, richer, healthier and living in more affluent areas were more satisfied with life. Blacks, Chinese and others were less satisfied than whites. Again, there is no significant difference between people in different class positions in this respect.

Descriptive data on health is not presented but a brief summary is in place here. There are notable differences between classes, with 53.6 per cent of the service class as against 36.5 per cent of the working class reporting excellent/very good health. Ethnic differences in self-reported health are also pronounced. Overall, 45.3 per cent of our respondents reported excellent/very good health but the proportions for Indians and Pakistanis/Bangladeshis were only 33.2 and 30.9 per cent respectively.

The brief analysis above suggests complicated interrelations between socioeconomic conditions, social capital and wellbeing, which cannot be unravelled in the bivariate analysis. Statistical modelling is needed to tackle the complexities.

Table 6.3 Ordinal logit regression coefficients on reported general health by social capital dimensions and sociodemographic attributes

	Model 1	Model 2	Model 3
Neighbourhood attachment	-0.023[†]	0.033[**]	0.048[***]
Social network	0.101[***]	0.071[***]	0.062[***]
Civic participation	0.139[***]	0.206[***]	0.094[***]
Age/10		-0.239[**]	-0.477[***]
Age squared/100		-0.002	0.035[***]
Sex			
Male		0.188[***]	0.096[†]
Female (base)			
Marital status			
Married		0.193[**]	0.099
Single		0.019	0.014
Divorced/separated/widowed (base)			
Ethnicity			
White (base)			
Black		0.005	0.216
Indian		-0.603[***]	-0.581[***]
Pakistani/Bangladeshi		-0.993[**]	-0.325
Chinese/other		-0.030	0.029
Employment status			
Employed			0.312[*]
Non-employed			-0.135
Unemployed (base)			
Class			
Service class			0.311[***]
Intermediate			0.298[***]
Working class (base)			

	Model 1	Model 2	Model 3
Education			
Tertiary			0.347***
Secondary			0.377***
Primary/none (base)			
Income			
Top quartile			0.491***
2nd			0.420***
3rd			0.304***
Bottom (base)			
Social deprivation			
Affluent areas			0.188**
Middle			0.065
Deprived areas (base)			
Intercept 1	-1.341	-2.333	-1.712
Intercept 2	0.192	0.729	-0.024
Pseudo R^2	0.012	0.038	0.059
N	7187	7128	6799

†$p<0.10$, *$p<0.05$, **$p<0.01$ and ***$p<0.001$

Note: Owing to the amount of data presented, standard errors and the 95% confidence intervals are not shown but are available on request.

Table 6.3 presents three models of ordinal logit regression on health (coded as 1 = fair/ poor, 2 = good, 3 = excellent/very good, so higher values of the coefficients in the form of log odds would mean better health). In Model 1, only the three dimensions of social capital are included; in Model 2, demographic attributes are added of age, sex, marital status and ethnicity; and in Model 3, socioeconomic factors are further added – employment status, class, education, standardized household mean income in quartiles and ward-level social deprivation.

The data in Model 1 of Table 6.3 show that people with higher levels of neighbourhood attachment at Wave 7 were less likely to report good health in Wave 9, but having stronger social network and civic engagement scores was positively associated with good heath status two years later. This, as noted earlier, could be due to confounding factors. As poorly educated working class respondents in poor financial situations tend to have higher scores in neighbourhood attachment (Li *et al.* 2005: Table 2), controlling for these factors might change the patterns (for discussions of policy initiatives to strengthen neighbourhood and regions for health improvement, see in particular Chapters 12 and 14). In Model 2, when the demographic attributes are added, it is noted that the negative association between neighbourhood attachment and health does now turn positive. Ethnic minority groups, particularly blacks, were likely to have lower scores in neighbourhood attachment (Li 2005), but blacks with similar levels of neighbourhood attachment were no less healthy. Indians, Pakistanis and Bangladeshis were found to be less healthy. With these factors controlled for, neighbourhood attachment is now positively associated with health. Men and the married tend to have better health and older people tend to have worse health, confirming other research findings (Helliwell and Putnam 2004).

Finally, in Model 3, further variables are added: on employment, class, education, income and ward-level deprivation. Comparing the coefficients between Models 2 and 3, it is found that the coefficients for neighbourhood attachment went up while those for social network and civic participation went down, suggesting that, other things being equal, maintaining good neighbourly relations would, as Putnam (2000) suggests, enhance health. On the other hand, gender, marital and some of the ethnic differences were much weakened or disappeared. With social capital and demographic factors controlled for, it was also found, as would be expected, that people who were employed, in higher class and educational positions, having higher family incomes and resident in more affluent areas would report better health. For present purposes, the most important finding is that social capital does appear to have independent and positive effects on people's perceived health.

Table 6.4 OLS regression coefficients on reported subjective wellbeing by social capital dimensions and sociodemographic attributes

	Model 1	Model 2	Model 3	Model 4
Neighbourhood attachment	0.154***	0.233***	0.235***	0.202***
Social network	0.259***	0.276***	0.262***	0.210***
Civic participation	0.020	0.056	0.006	-0.073
Age/10		-0.564*	-0.845**	-0.448†
Age squared/100		0.052*	0.096***	0.066**
Sex				
Male		1.673***	1.522***	1.438***
Female (base)				
Marital status				
Married		0.254	0.140	0.065
Single		0.689**	0.645*	0.622*
Divorced/separated/widowed (base)				
Ethnicity				
White (base)				
Black		0.615	0.518	0.372
Indian		-0.732	-0.454	-0.089
Pakistani/Bangladeshi		-0.100	0.284	0.293
Chinese/other		-0.227	0.245	0.258
Employment status				
Employed			0.634	0.454
Non-employed			0.094	0.361
Unemployed (base)				
Class				
Service class			-0.236	-0.506**
Intermediate			-0.127	-0.391*
Working class (base)				
Education				
Tertiary			0.199	-0.121
Secondary			0.245	-0.099
Primary/none (base)				
Income				
Top quartile			0.942***	0.474*

	Model 1	Model 2	Model 3	Model 4
2nd			1.083***	0.666***
3rd			0.789***	0.522*
Bottom (base)				
Social deprivation				
Affluent areas			0.088	-0.135
Middle			0.033	-0.070
Deprived areas (base)				
Health				
Excellent/very good				4.714***
Good				3.502***
Fair/poor (base)				
Constant	24.998***	25.208***	24.369***	20.846***
R^2	0.021	0.052	0.060	0.159
N	7,062	7,005	6,685	6,684

†$p<0.10$, *$p<0.05$, **$p<0.01$ and ***$p<0.001$

Table 6.5 OLS regression coefficients on reported overall satisfaction with life by social capital dimensions and sociodemographic attributes

	Model 1	Model 2	Model 3	Model 4
Neighbourhood attachment	0.097***	0.085***	0.088***	0.080***
Social network	0.071***	0.082***	0.077***	0.066***
Civic participation	0.023	0.004	-0.008	-0.026†
Age/10		-0.269***	-0.366***	-0.271***
Age squared/100		0.034***	0.046***	0.039***
Sex				
Male		0.116***	0.091**	0.072*
Female (base)				
Marital status				
Married		0.365***	0.331***	0.311***
Single		0.216***	0.207**	0.197**
Divorced/separated/widowed (base)				
Ethnicity				
White (base)				
Black		-0.188	-0.134	-0.172
Indian		-0.252	-0.218	-0.130
Pakistani/Bangladeshi		-0.062	0.073	0.081
Chinese/other		-0.286	-0.153	-0.170
Employment status				
Employed			0.394***	0.337**
Non-employed			0.272*	0.320**
Unemployed (base)				
Class				
Service class			-0.034	-0.097*
Intermediate			-0.024	-0.085*
Working class (base)				
Education				
Tertiary			-0.103*	-0.180***
Secondary			-0.082†	-0.165***

	Model 1	Model 2	Model 3	Model 4
Primary/none (base)				
Income				
Top quartile			0.362^{***}	0.258^{***}
2nd			0.255^{***}	0.163^{**}
3rd			0.159^{**}	$0.100^{\dagger}$
Bottom (base)				
Social deprivation				
Affluent areas			0.016	-0.035
Middle			0.030	0.005
Deprived areas (base)				
Health				
Excellent/very good				1.089^{***}
Good				0.777^{***}
Fair/poor (base)				
Constant	5.223^{***}	5.312^{***}	5.020^{***}	4.229^{***}
R^2	0.053	0.076	0.091	0.192
N	7,094	7,038	6,715	6,714

$^{\dagger}p<0.10$, $^{*}p<0.05$, $^{**}p<0.01$ and $^{***}p<0.001$

Tables 6.4 and 6.5 present ordinary least squares estimation (OLS) regression analysis on happiness and life satisfaction respectively, each with four models. The first three models have the same structure as that in Table 6.3 and, in Model 4, health status is further included as a control. The purpose is to see whether the three types of social capital as have been conceptualized and measured would still have significant impacts on happiness and life satisfaction with the progressive inclusion of demographic, socio-cultural and health factors.

With regard to happiness data, it was found, in Model 1 of Table 6.4, that higher levels of informal social capital at Waves 7 and 8, namely neighbourhood attachment and social network, are significantly associated with greater happiness at Wave 9, while there is no significant association between civic engagement and happiness. When the coefficients are compared from Model 1, where only social capital types are included, to those in Models 2, 3 and 4, where more variables are progressively included, it is found that informal social capital measures remain highly significant in each model. The patterns here suggest that having stronger social ties with friends and neighbours does enhance people's sense of happiness over and above other factors.

The other patterns in the tables generally confirm findings in existing studies. Thus older people tend to be less happy, but after a certain age happiness will increase (Blanchflower and Oswald 2004). Men consistently reported greater happiness than women. The never married single were happier than the once married – that is, those who were separated, or divorced, or widowed. It is interesting to note that the married were found to be significantly happier in the bivariate analysis in Table 6.2 but not so in the multivariate analysis here. The reason may be that, as Putnam (2000) argues, marriage is a form of social capital itself in that married people tend to have greater access to and stronger social ties with extended kin, neighbours, friends and spouse's colleagues and friends. Married people also tend to have higher personal earnings and family incomes (Chun and Lee 2001). Most important of all, the once married were predominantly women (71 per cent). Thus when all these factors were controlled for, marriage effects were much reduced or disappeared. Health status is, as expected, a crucial predictor of happiness. Other things being equal, women in service class jobs were more distressed, for such jobs were psychologically more demanding and they also carried the dual burden. With all other factors in the models controlled for, ethnicity, employment status, levels of education and local ward-level social deprivation did not affect happiness.

The data on life satisfaction in Table 6.5 can be summarized in brief as the patterns are rather similar to those on happiness. In particular, positive effects of informal social capital, curvilinear effects of age, and pronounced effects of income and health are found. The major differences between patterns in the two tables lie in the fact that while the married were not significantly happier than the once married, or the employed than the unemployed, they were found to be more satisfied with life overall. The likely reason for this discrepancy is, as Helliwell and Putnam (2004) explain, that happiness self-estimation reflects a more short-term, situation-dependent, mood, while life satisfaction self-estimation reflects a more enduring, stable, longer-term evaluation. Other things being equal, married people in employment were much more satisfied with life than being merely happy.

Finally, it is interesting to note the few apparently surprising results with regard to happiness and life satisfaction. First, health has a much more pronounced effect on happiness than on life satisfaction (4.714 and 1.089 respectively for excellent/very good versus fair/poor health: Tables 6.4 and 6.5). This difference in magnitude is due to the different scales of the two measures used: happiness ranging from 0 to 36 and life satisfaction from 1 to 7. If standardized scores were used, the effects would be similar, 0.447 and 0.428 respectively. Second, service class members were found to be less happy and less satisfied with life, as were the highly educated with life satisfaction. On the face of it, the results here are odd. It is known that the service class and the highly educated are less likely to be unemployed. They are also more likely to earn much more, to live in more affluent areas and to enjoy better health, which are all essential elements for happiness and life satisfaction. Why, then, were they less happy and less satisfied? The answer is that the service class is being compared to the working class, all other things being equal. Since the two classes are not equal in job security, income, health or local affluence, further analysis made the oddities disappear. Thus the service class respondents with higher incomes or in better health were not significantly more unhappy or dissatisfied than their working-class counterparts; if anything, service class respondents in better health status were found significantly more satisfied with life. Nor were the highly educated who were working, with higher incomes or in better health found less dissatisfied (on the changing dynamics of social class in relation to health, see in particular Chapter 4).

It has been shown that it is possible to develop measures of social capital based on theoretical insights, particularly those by Putnam (2000), and to use these measures in the analysis of subjective wellbeing. The adopted research design made use of the longitudinal nature of the BHPS data, which is a step forward in this area of research where most studies are based on cross-sectional data.

Analysis shows some important findings. First, as social capital theorists, with limited data support, have constantly suggested, higher levels of social capital, particularly those in the form of informal social networks with neighbours and friends, do appear to enhance people's healthiness, happiness and perceived life satisfaction, and this is the case even when most of the sociologically important independent variables at both individual and contextual levels are taken into account. Thus, even though social capital is socially skewed in favour of those in more advantaged socioeconomic positions (Li *et al.* 2003, 2005, 2006) it also has an independent role to play in people's physical and mental health over and above the sociocultural resources. All this lends support to the social capital project, and gives credence to the distinction between formal and informal social capital and to the greater weight placed on the informal kind as Putnam (2000) argues (for the implications of strengthening social capital in health policy whether through neighbourhoods, regions or family support, see in particular Chapters 12, 13, 14 and 16).

Second, findings also support the idea that life satisfaction is a more enduring, future oriented property than happiness. This is reflected in the stronger association of marriage and employment status with life satisfaction (Table 6.5) than with happiness (Table 6.4). For most people, these are the two most important pillars of life: avoiding unemployment in the public arena and having a happy conjugal family life in the domestic sphere (on the changing demographics of partnership as distinct from marriage, see Chapter 3).

Apart from these, some findings emerge which cannot easily be explained. Respondents of Indian ethnicity are less likely than the whites to report top health status (excellent/very good) even when they are in the top income quartiles (Table 6.4). The data do not allow for further analysis in this regard but two hypotheses are offered for possible future exploration. First, there may be something in the culture and tradition that makes respondents of Indian ethnicity more reserved in making responses. What passes as excellent/very good health for a person recorded as white might be regarded as good for a person recorded as Indian. Thus, in the 2001 census of the population and in the General Household Survey (GHS) of 2001 where only 'good, fair, poor' health were asked of the respondents, Indians were no less than whites in recording good health (65.6 and 62.4 per cent for Indians and whites in the census, and 60.3 and 59.1 per cent for the two groups in the GHS, respectively). Second, social capital might help raise greater awareness of health issues among people of Indian ethnicity. According to the 2001 census, there are more health professionals among Indians (3.99 per cent) than among any other ethnic group (0.49 for whites and 0.66 for England and Wales as a whole). On average, Indians have more co-ethnic medical experts among their social networks than do any other ethnic group, giving them more chances to exchange health-related information and making them more knowledgeable of health issues. What passes unnoticed for other ethnic groups might, for people recording Indian ethnicity, be viewed as something of a health concern. While these might offer channels for future exploration, analysis does not indicate that Indians are at any health disadvantage.

References

Argyle, M. (1989) *The Psychology of Happiness*. London: Routledge.

Blanchflower, D. and Oswald, A. (2004) Wellbeing over time in Britain and the USA, *Journal of Public Economics*, 88(7–8): 1359–86.

Bourdieu, P. (1984) *Distinction: A Social Critique of the Judgment of Taste*, translated by Richard Nice. London: Routledge & Kegan Paul.

Bourdieu, P. (1986) The forms of capital, in J. Westport (ed.) *Handbook of Theory and Research for the Sociology of Education*. New York: Greenwood.

Bourdieu, P. and Wacquant, L. (1992) *An Invitation to Reflexive Sociology*. Chicago: Chicago University Press.

Buck, N. (2000) Housing, location and residential mobility, in R. Berthoud and J. Gershuny (eds) *Seven Years in the Lives of British Families*. Bristol: The Policy Press.

Burt, R. (1992) *Structural Holes*. Cambridge, MA: Harvard University Press.

Burt, R. (2000) The network structure of social capital, *Research in Organisational Behaviour*, 22: 345–423.

Carstairs, V. and Morris, R. (1989) Deprivation, mortality and resource allocation, *Community Medicine*, 11(4): 364–72.

Chandola, T., Wiggins, R., Schofield, P. and Bartley, M. (2003) Social inequalities in health by individual and household measures of social position in a cohort of healthy people, *Journal of Epidemiology and Community Health*, 57: 56–62.

Chun, H. and Lee, I. (2001) Why do married men earn more: productivity or marriage selection? *Economic Inquiry*, 39(2): 307–19.

Coleman, J.S. (1988) Social capital in the creation of human capital, *American Journal of Sociology*, 94: S95–120.

Coleman, J.S. (1990) *Foundations of Social Theory*. Cambridge, MA: Harvard University Press.

Edwards, M. (2004) *Civil Society*. Cambridge: Polity.

Field, J. (2003) *Social Capital*. London: Routledge.

Fine, B. (2001) *Social Capital versus Social Theory: Political Economy and Social Science at the Turn of the Millennium*. London: Routledge.

Gardner, J. and Oswald, A. (2006) Do divorcing couples become happier by breaking up? *Journal of the Royal Statistical Society*, 169(2): 319–36.

Goldthorpe, J.H. with Llewellyn, C. and Payne, C. (1987) *Social Mobility and Class Structure in Modern Britain*. Oxford: Clarendon Press.

Granovetter, M.S. (1973) The strength of weak ties, *American Journal of Sociology*, 78(6): 1360–80.

Granovetter, M.S. (1974) *Getting a Job: A Study of Contacts and Careers*. Cambridge, MA: Harvard University Press.

Granovetter, M.S. (1985) Economic action and social structure: the problem of embeddedness, *American Journal of Sociology*, 91: 481–510.

Hall, P. (1999) Social capital in Britain, *British Journal of Political Science*, 29: 417–61.

Helliwell, J.F. and Putnam, R.D. (2004) The social context of wellbeing, *Philosophical Transactions of the Royal Society*, 359: 1435–46.

Hertzman, C., Power, C., Matthews, S. and Manor, O. (2001) Using an interactive framework of society and lifecourse to explain self-rated health in early adulthood, *Social Science & Medicine*, 53: 1575–85.

Jenkins, S.P. (1999) *Modelling Household Income Dynamics*. ISER Working Paper.

Kadushin, C. (2004) Too much investment in social capital? *Social Networks*, 26: 75–90.

Karn, V. (ed.) (1997) *Ethnicity in the 1991 Census*, Vol. 4. London: The Stationery Office.

Kawachi, I., Kennedy, B., Lochner, K. and Prothrow-Stith, D. (1997) Social capital, income inequality and mortality, *American Journal of Public Health*, 87(9): 1491–8.

Keane, J. (1998) *Civil Society*. Cambridge: Polity Press.

Li, Y. (2005) Social capital, ethnicity and the labour market, *Proceedings on Engaging Community*, http://engagingcommunities2005.org/abstracts/Li-Yaojun-final.pdf.

Li, Y., Bechhofer, F., McCrone, D., Anderson, M. and Stewart, R. (2002) A divided working class? Planning and career perception in the service and working classes, *Work, Employment and Society*, 16(4): 617–36.

Li, Y., Savage, M. and Pickles, A. (2003) Social capital and social exclusion in England and Wales (1972–1999), *British Journal of Sociology*, 54(4): 497–526.

Li, Y., Pickles, A. and Savage, M. (2005) Social capital and social trust in Britain, *European Sociological Review*, 21(2): 109–23.

Li, Y., Savage, M. and Warde, A. (2006) Informal connections, civic engagement and social capital in the UK: a new analysis. Mimeo: Birmingham University.

Lin, N. (1999a) Inequality in social capital, *Contemporary Sociology*, 29(6): 785–95.

Lin, N. (1999b) Social networks and status attainment, *Annual Review of Sociology*, 25: 467–87.

Lin, N. (2001) *Social Capital*. Cambridge: Cambridge University Press.

Lin, N., Ensel, W.M. and Vaughn, J.C. (1981) Social resources and the strength of ties: structural factors in occupational attainment, *American Sociological Review*, 46: 393–405.

Lin, N., Ye, X. and Ensel, W. (1999) Social support and depressed mood: A structural analysis, *Journal of Health and Social Behaviour*, 40(4): 344–59.

Modood, T. and Berthoud, R. (1997) *Ethnic Minorities in Britain: Diversity and Disadvantage*. London: Policy Studies Institute.

Paxton, P. (1999) Is social capital declining in the United States? A multiple indicator assessment, *American Journal of Sociology*, 105(1): 88–127.

Pevalin, D. (2000) Multiple applications of the GHQ-12 in a general population sample: an investigation of long-term retest effects, *Social Psychiatry and Psychiatric Epidemiology*, 35(11): 508–12.

Pevalin, D. and Rose, D. (2003) *Social Capital for Health*. London: Health Development Agency.

Putnam, R. (1993) *Making Democracy Work: Civic Traditions in Modern Italy*. Princeton, NJ: Princeton University Press.

Putnam, R. (2000) *Bowling Alone: The Collapse and Revival of American Community*. New York: Simon & Schuster.

Ross, C. and Wu, C. (1995) The links between education and health, *American Sociological Review*, 60(5): 719–45.

Schwartz, S. (1994) The fallacy of the ecological fallacy: the potential misuse of a concept and the consequences, *American Journal of Public Health*, 84: 819–24.

Shields, M.A. and Wheatley Price, S. (2005) Exploring the economic and social determinants of psychological wellbeing and perceived social support in England, *Journal of the Royal Statistical Society A*, 168(3): 513–37.

Skocpol, T. (1996) Unravelling from above, *American Prospect*, 25: 20–5.

Stutzer, A. and Frey, B. (2006) Does marriage make people happy, or do happy people get married? *The Journal of Socio-Economics*, 35: 326–47.

Taylor, M., Brice, J., Buck, N. and Prentice-Lane, E. (2002) *British Household Panel Survey User Manual*. Colchester: University of Essex.

White, A. (2002) *Social Focus in Brief: Ethnicity 2002*. London: Office for National Statistics.

Wilkinson, R. (2002) Liberty, fraternity, equality, *International Journal of Epidemiology*, 31: 538–43.

Wilson, W. (1967) Correlates of avowed happiness, *Psychological Bulletin*, 67: 294–306.

7 Ethnicity and racism in the politics of health

Hannah Bradby and Tarani Chandola

Ethnicity has multiple meanings. While genetics and racism are part of what is encompassed by the term ethnicity, its current meanings are primarily associated with identity and especially aspects of identity which are cultural and where there is some measure of voluntarism in their adoption. Ethnicity is sometimes contrasted with race, with the latter assumed to be a biological category over which the individual has little control. Thus ethnicity is taken to refer to all those aspects of group based identity which do not rest on genetic difference. However, this version of ethnicity as cultural identity is contested by those who suggest that the way the term is used shows that it is simply a euphemism for race. Using ethnicity to avoid the word race is problematic if a belief in a biological and immutable categoric disjuncture in humanity is thereby left unchallenged. Where ethnicity is misused to refer to the effects of racism, that is to say discrimination based on a belief in the reality of biological categories of race, this can imply that inequalities are due to the culture of the minority rather than the way that a minority is treated by others. Euphemisms are unhelpful in any analytic discourse and are particularly problematic here, given that conceptual clarity around the target of a public health intervention is crucial if attempting to make policy to remedy inequalities. Disputes over the status of race as a scientific, sociological and ethical concept have been fraught (Bradby 2003), with some scholars believing that reproducing race as a research variable inscribes oppressive categories. An assimilationist assumption, that once immigrants have lived in the UK for a generation they will take on the ways of the majority and become culturally indistinguishable (Mason 2000), has been combined with a general reluctance to draw attention to racialized divisions in Britain.

Ethnicity as migrant status

In high-income states ethnicity has come to be regarded as a characteristic of minority groups, usually those established as a result of migration motivated either by a search for work or flight from an oppressive regime, or in the case of states with a history of mass slavery, migration that is coerced. The arrival of new groups, distinguished by their language, religion and habits of dress and diet has long been a feature of British life, particularly in big cities which offer employment and trading opportunities, and ports with significant maritime traffic.

Previous waves of migrants from continental Europe and Ireland are sometimes perceived as having been absorbed into the British population with some degree of invisibility in public policy terms. Thus the presumption that migrant populations will take on a British way of life, thereby assuming the health risks and benefits of the general population, tended to remain unchallenged until recently. The labour migration after the Second World War from the Indian subcontinent and the Caribbean gave rise to minorities who were visible and who maintained a distinct cultural life. Whether or not previous waves of migration, such as the Catholic Irish escaping from famine and continental European Jews fleeing anti-Semitism, really did assimilate, any non-assimilation or cultural incompatibility with the majority has tended not to feature recently as a public health problem, although it did so for previous generations (see for example Maglen 2005 and Wray 2006 on the health background to the 1905 Aliens Act in Britain). Of course public perceptions may be very different from the felt experience, as in the case of the Irish in Britain, particularly Irish men, whose health has been poorer than that of the host populations (see for example Bracken *et al.* 1998; Leavey 1999; DoH 2001; Walls and Williams 2004).

A general feature of work on migrant health inequalities has been the excessive attention given to relative risks of specific conditions, rather than assessing absolute risks that might better reflect the overall health of the whole minority population (Smaje 1995: 35). Nonetheless, using mortality as an indicator of health, overall rates in England and Wales, since statistics for Scotland and Northern Ireland being gathered separately, were lower compared with the migrants' place of birth, but higher than for the resident population (Marmot *et al.* 1984; Balarajan and Balusu 1990). Attempts to control for the confounding effect of class among migrants led to the conclusion that differences in the social class distribution of mortality were not the explanation of the different mortality of immigrants from one another and compared to the general population (Marmot *et al.* 1984). A unitary theory of raised levels of mortality for migrants was always unlikely given the enormous contrasts between the cultures and migration histories of migrants from countries showing health penalties, for example, Ireland and Pakistan (Smaje 1995). Smaje regrets the dearth of work considering migrants' general health, and the bias towards studies of the use of particular services, especially reproductive and mental health services, and the experience of particular conditions. Surveys of minority populations across a range of common health conditions showed that coronary heart disease rates were raised for those born in the Indian subcontinent (Balarajan and Balusu 1990; Knight *et al.* 1993) and, in common with people born in Ireland, the gap with the general population was not closing.

In the 1990s questions of how to measure ethnicity, rather than simply migrant status, became more urgent as third and fourth generations of descendants of migrants could no longer be identified using country of birth or parents' country of birth. The question of whether country of birth constituted a suitable proxy for a broader, more complex notion of ethnicity had remained largely unexplored. But with researchers seeking to define health outcomes among the grandchildren and great grandchildren of migrants, the discussion reopened and the contested nature of ethnicity became apparent (Bradby 1995; Nazroo 1998).

Ethnicity as genetics

The difficulties in defining ethnicity correspond to the problems in measuring it. Throughout the twentieth century assumed phenotypically based concepts of race were being challenged. After the Second World War the ghastly implications of Nazi racist policies became clear and gradually the relegation of people to a subservient class based on ethnic group or race has become more difficult to maintain in countries that claimed to be democratic: segregation became illegal in the USA during the 1950s and minority white rule with apartheid was dismantled in South Africa during the 1990s. The idea that humanity could be divided up into distinct groups and hierarchically ordered has been shown to be an oppressive ideology rather than an empirically observed scientific truth. The assumption that health differences between culture groups can be attributed to underlying genetic differences between populations has been demonstrated to be fallacious.

Variation within ethnic groups

It was with the publication of the results from the *Fourth National Survey of Ethnic Minorities*, conducted by the Policy Studies Institute, that the debate really matured in the UK. This survey included, for the first time, an extensive section on health, health-related behaviours and the use of health services, and was able to explore the complex relationship between health and ethnicity using a sample that was fully representative of the ethnic groups included (Modood *et al.* 1997). The recorded detail on the lives of members of different ethnic groups also meant that factors that might explain the relationship between ethnicity and health could be directly considered. The report challenged current assumptions about the uniform pattern of ill health across broadly defined ethnic groups, such as South Asian. It also illustrated the importance of socioeconomic factors to ethnic differences in health, both within particular ethnic groups and when making comparisons across ethnic groups (Nazroo 1997).

Statutory data-gathering requirements

Problems of measuring ethnicity, especially in statutory statistics, have been the focus of much discussion (Aspinall 2000). The 2001 UK census question set on ethnicity included a substantially revised ethnic group question and a new question on religion which addressed some of the shortcomings in the 1991 census question on ethnicity. However, Aspinall (2000) argues that there remain problems with the lack of detail on the ethnic origins of the 'white' group, including those of Irish and Scottish origin, as well as the use of Indian subcontinent groups, that ignores important differences between religious and linguistic communities within the broad categories of Indian, Pakistani and Bangladeshi. Despite these problems in measurement, a proposal has been made to include ethnicity at birth and death registration in England and Wales (Aspinall *et al.* 2003).

Data from the 2001 census shows that 87 per cent of the population of England and

96 per cent of the population of Wales gave their ethnic origin as white British with other white categories making up the largest minorities. In Scotland, 88 per cent of the population gave their ethnic origin as white Scottish and a further 10 per cent as some other white origin, including Irish. People who give their origins as Pakistani make up 2.9 per cent of the population of England and Wales and 0.63 per cent of the Scottish population, with people of Indian origin making up 2 per cent of the population of England and Wales and 0.3 per cent of the population in Scotland. In Northern Ireland more than 99 per cent of those responding in the 2001 census gave their ethnic group as white. The total number of people from minority ethnic groups grew from 6 to 9 per cent of the population between 1991 and 2001 according to the census data for England and Wales, partly due to the addition of a 'mixed' category. People from minority groups are clustered in London, which has the highest proportion of all minorities except for people of Pakistani origin, whose greatest concentration is in the West Midlands and Yorkshire and Humber. But even in local areas with the highest concentration of a single minority, they remain minorities. For instance, 33 per cent of people in Tower Hamlets are of Bangladeshi origin and 26 per cent of people in Leicester are of Indian origin.

All public authorities in the UK listed under the Race Relations (Amendment) Act 2000 have a general duty to promote race equality. This includes the standard collection and use of ethnic group and related data on patients, service users and staff of the National Health Service (NHS) and social services. However, data from the Hospital Episode Statistics for England in 2002–3 show that only 68.1 per cent of all hospital episodes had a valid ethnic group coding (Aspinall and Jacobson 2004). In addition to incompleteness, there may also be problems with data quality as some hospital trusts are still using the 1991 census classification to identify ethnic groups and others assign ethnicity on the basis of staff observation rather than patient self identification (Aspinall and Jacobson 2004).

Patterns of ethnicity and health from the Health Survey for England

Since the Fourth National Survey, there have been two large-scale surveys of adults and children, representative of minority ethnic groups across England: the Health Surveys for England in 1999 (DoH 2001; Erens *et al.* 2001) and in 2004 (DoH 2005; Sproston and Mindell 2006). In addition to self-reported information, objective physical measurements and blood, urine and saliva samples were analysed. Both surveys reveal a complex distribution of these indicators among the major ethnic groups (for further discussion of wellbeing, social capital and health in relation to ethnicity, see Chapter 6).

In 1999, among men, the prevalence of limiting long-standing illness was between 30 and 65 per cent higher for Pakistani, Bangladeshi and Irish men than for men in the general population (DoH 2001). Among women, black Caribbean and South Asian groups were between 20 and 45 per cent more likely to report limiting long-standing illness than women in the general population. Chinese adults in contrast were about 40 per cent less likely than the general population, and less than all other minority ethnic groups, to report limiting long standing illness. By 2004, the levels of long-standing illness and limiting long standing illness were significantly higher for Pakistani women than they were in 1999, whereas for Indian women, the levels in 2004 were significantly lower (DoH 2005).

In 1999, Pakistani and Bangladeshi men and women had significantly higher rates of cardiovascular disease (CVD) than the general population, while Chinese men and women had lower rates (DoH 2001). The prevalence of CVD was also higher among black Caribbean women. By 2004, the prevalence of CVD had doubled among Pakistani men and Indian women (DoH 2005). In 1999 and in 2004, South Asian (Indian, Pakistani and Bangladeshi) men and women had the highest rates of diabetes. Rates of diabetes among the black Caribbean population were also significantly higher than in the general population.

In terms of communicable diseases, tuberculosis and sexually transmitted infections are distributed differentially across ethnic groups. In 2001, the highest tuberculosis rate was found among black Africans (211 per 100,000), followed by Pakistani (145 per 100,000), Indian (104 per 100,000) and Bangladeshi groups (62 per 100,000) (Aspinall and Jacobson 2004). In comparison the tuberculosis rate for white groups is 4 per 100,000 population. HIV and sexually transmitted infections also disproportionately affect black and minority ethnic groups in the UK. Furthermore, undiagnosed HIV infection and late diagnosis is more common among some minority ethnic groups.

Mental health

In 1999, Bangladeshi and Pakistani men and women were more likely than the general population to suffer from minor psychiatric morbidity, measured by the 12-item General Health Questionnaire (GHQ-12), as were black Caribbean and Indian women, while Chinese men and women were far less likely to have minor psychiatric morbidity (DoH 2001). Among black Caribbean and Indian men, and Irish men and women, the prevalence of high GHQ-12 scores did not differ from the general population. The prevalence of minor psychiatric morbidity was lower in 2004 in the general population and among Irish and Bangladeshi men and women, and black Caribbean and Indian women when compared with 1999 data (DoH 2005). For Chinese men, in contrast, the prevalence was higher in 2004 than it had been in 1999.

As the research from the Health Survey for England suggests, there are differences in mental health across ethnic groups. However, these results are not congruent with two key findings in the literature on ethnicity and mental health in the UK, namely the apparently high rates of schizophrenia and other forms of psychosis among African-Caribbean people, and the apparently low rates of mental illness generally among South Asian people (Cochrane and Bal 1989). The literature on ethnic differences in psychotic illnesses suggests that rates of first contact with treatment services for such illnesses are three to five times higher for black Caribbean people than the general population.

In order to address this controversial area, the Ethnic Minority Psychiatric Illness Rates in the Community (EMPIRIC) study was conducted. It comprised a quantitative survey of rates of mental illness among different ethnic groups in England and a qualitative study investigating ethnic and cultural differences in the context, experience and expression of mental distress (Joint Health Surveys Unit 2002). This report highlighted a major weakness of most work on ethnicity and mental illness, which tends to rely on data based on contact with treatment services. Contact with services, even when access is universal, as in the NHS, reflects illness behaviour rather than illness per se (Blane *et al.* 1996). This makes interpreting differences in treatment rates across ethnic groups difficult, particularly as illness behaviour is likely to be influenced by a number of factors that are influenced by ethnicity, such as socioeconomic position, health beliefs, expectations of the sick role and lay referral systems. In contrast to studies on rates of contact with services, the EMPIRIC study indicated a twofold higher rate for black Caribbean people compared with the white group. This difference was not significant for men or the total black Caribbean population and was not significant at the level of estimated rates of psychosis. Even if black Caribbean people are more vulnerable to psychotic illnesses, the discrepancy between the data from psychiatric services and the general population suggests that they are also treated differently in the UK. Possible explanations suggested by EMPIRIC are racism by psychiatrists and in the community, misunderstanding of cultural expressions of distress, differential responses by police, social and treatment services, and social inequality. However, why such factors should operate for black Caribbean people as opposed to other ethnic minorities is not clear.

Factors associated with ethnic differences in health

The Fourth National Survey illustrated the importance of socioeconomic factors in understanding the pattern of ethnic differences in health (Nazroo 1997). This pattern of socioeconomic disadvantage is often multidimensional, reflecting the poorer living conditions of many ethnic minorities in terms of housing or neighbourhood conditions, underemployment and unemployment (Chandola 2001). In addition, other factors such as differences in health behaviours, access to health services and the experience of racial discrimination have also been highlighted as contributing towards this pattern.

Behavioural risk factors

The distribution of health behaviours among different ethnic groups is complex. Some of these differences may be affected by cultural patterns of traditional diet and lifestyle; others may arise due to the differential rate of change in the behavioural patterns of the general population compared to ethnic minority groups. So for example, chewing tobacco products such as *paan* mixed with tobacco is common to some of the South Asian groups. In 1999, Bangladeshi and Irish men reported using tobacco products much more than the general population (DoH 2001). Although Bangladeshi women were similar to the general population in terms of self-reported tobacco use, they had a much higher risk of a saliva cotinine level of 15 ng/ml or over than any other group of women. Saliva cotinine levels are an indicator of actual tobacco use. Black Caribbean, Bangladeshi and Irish men in 1999 had a higher proportion of smokers compared with the general population. By 2001, the prevalence of cigarette smoking was highest among Bangladeshi, Irish and Pakistani men (DoH 2001). While the smoking rates of Irish men had fallen considerably, the higher prevalence for Bangladeshi and Pakistani men and the high use of tobacco products among Bangladeshi women is a matter of some public health concern.

Obesity, a major risk factor for cardiovascular disease, is increasing worldwide and the causes of this increase are much debated (for further discussion, see Chapter 3). Some of the explanations look at the imbalance between physical activity or energy output and diet or energy intake. The distribution of obesity among ethnic groups in England is different depending on the measurement of obesity chosen. In terms of body mass index, black African, Pakistani and black Caribbean women tend to be more overweight than the general female population, while in terms of raised waist-hip ratio, Pakistani and Bangladeshi men have a higher risk than the general male population (DoH 2005). Explanations for the raised risk of obesity for some ethnic minorities are probably not found in differences in dietary behaviour, as most ethnic minorities report healthier diets compared to the general population, whether in terms of consuming five or more portions of fruit and vegetables, or in terms of lower fat intake. Except for the Irish, whose behaviour replicates that of the general population, men and women from all minority ethnic groups report less alcohol consumption than is normal. This pattern has changed little between 1999 and 2004. However, in terms of physical activity, Indian, Pakistani, Bangladeshi and Chinese men and women are less likely to meet current recommended levels of activity compared with the general population. Between 1999 and 2004, this gap in physical activity increased for Indian, Pakistani and Bangladeshi men, and for Pakistani, Bangladeshi and Chinese women (DoH 2005).

Cigarette smoking, the use of tobacco products and lower physical activity levels are important risk factors for a range of health problems later on in life. Their higher prevalence, particularly in Bangladeshi and Pakistani groups, suggests that ethnic differences in health may continue to widen as men and women in these groups age (for more on the connection between smoking and ethnicity, see Chapters 10 and 17).

Racial discrimination

There are two main types of racial discrimination, interpersonal and institutional (Karlsen and Nazroo 2002). Interpersonal discrimination refers to discriminatory interactions between individuals, which usually can be directly perceived. Interpersonal discrimination has been shown to be associated with poorer health outcomes in the UK and USA, including physical and mental health outcomes, such as raised blood pressure, increased psychological distress, depression and poorer self-rated health (reviewed in Karlsen and Nazroo 2002). Reporting experiences of racial discrimination is also associated with increased prevalence of cigarette smoking.

Institutional discrimination typically refers to discriminatory policies or practices embedded in organizational structures and tends to be more invisible than interpersonal discrimination (Karlsen and Nazroo 2002). However, although people from ethnic minority groups have lower incomes and are concentrated in environmentally and economically poorer geographic areas, in poorer quality and more overcrowded accommodation, in less desirable occupations, and in longer periods of unemployment than their ethnic majority counterparts, there is little direct evidence on the extent to which the health disadvantage of ethnic minority groups is a product of institutional racism (for the effectiveness on health policies directed at locality, see Chapters 12 and 14; for a discussion of data on ethnicity and wellbeing, see Chapter 6).

Access to services

Access to health services is a key issue for marginalized minority ethnic groups, given the 'inverse care law' that those who need healthcare most are least likely to get it (Tudor-Hart 1971). However, as mentioned above, statistics on ethnicity are not always collected routinely by health service providers, and are often questionable in terms of accuracy of measurement.

The evidence suggests that differences in access to primary care may not be as important as access to secondary and community health services, and referrals to hospital services and treatments (Aspinall and Jacobson 2004). Survey evidence suggests that minority ethnic groups see their general practitioner as often or more than the general population. However, this does not translate into higher outpatient hospital attendance rates, which are lower for some minority ethnic groups. In terms of ethnic differences in hospital treatments, there is some evidence of inequity in specialist cardiac investigation services, especially for South Asian groups. Compared to the white population, South Asians with chronic chest pain may be less likely to be referred for exercise testing and wait longer to see a cardiologist or to have angiography (Lear *et al.* 1994). Feder *et al.* (2002) concluded that among patients deemed appropriate for coronary revascularization, South Asian patients are less likely to receive treatment compared with white patients. They also concluded that physician bias and socioeconomic factors did not explain these differences. A possible explanation could lie in the difference in the patient experiences of minority ethnic groups when negotiating health services.

The third National Survey of NHS patients (Airey *et al.* 1999) found that black and South Asian patients are more likely to report poorer patient experiences. They are more likely to report their appointment for their first treatment has been postponed or cancelled and longer waiting times for hospital treatment. South Asian groups, in particular, report poorer communication with health service providers, and often felt they were not always treated with dignity and respect. Non-insulin-dependent diabetes remains undiagnosed in up to 40 per cent of Asian diabetics. Several studies report inadequate quality of healthcare for Asian and African-Caribbean diabetics and poor compliance arising from patients' lack of knowledge about the disease and its management through inappropriate health information (Aspinall and Jacobson 2004).

There are a number of political and practical difficulties associated with the public health issues of minority ethnic groups. The range of ideas that the concept of ethnicity encompasses, including those of identity, origins and culture, means that its use in research and policy inevitably prioritizes some of these. In contemporary Britain self-assigned ethnicity has become the rule, although in some routine data collection ethnicity is still attributed by observation.

Research based on representative samples, including data on country of birth, religion, self-assigned ethnicity and experience of racism, has made it impossible to maintain any illusion that generalizations can be made about the health status of broadly defined ethnic groups. Variations by gender, between minorities and through time, have been documented which suggest that the challenge of documenting, let along remedying, health inequalities influenced by ethnicity, has only just begun. Poor health outcomes documented for particular minority ethnic groups cannot be attributed to a single factor such as gender, locality, racism or poverty, but stem from their interaction. The ill effects of poverty, racism and locality can compound one another. Given the complexity of these factors, the scope and utility for internationally recognized and shared categories of ethnicity remains in doubt.

Commentators have consistently pointed to the way that ethnicity is assumed to pertain to minorities rather than majorities. If ethnicity is a sociologically useful concept it should, logically, be equally applicable to evaluating the causes of the patterns of health of majorities. Logical analysis notwithstanding, ethnicity looks set to remain a means of describing minority culture, context and circumstance, with alternative variables being sought to explain the circumstances of general populations. The dynamic, contingent nature of cultural groupings means that even populations that show stable patterns of ethnicity should not be essentialized. Given that the fastest-growing ethnic group in Britain is made up of those who describe themselves as of mixed origins, the future picture is likely to differ from our current understanding.

References

Airey, C., Bruster, S., Erens, B., Lilley, S.J., Pickering, K. and Pitson, L. (1999) *National Surveys of NHS Patients: General Practice*. London: NHS Executive.

Aspinall, P. (2000) The new 2001 census question set on cultural characteristics: is it useful for the monitoring of the health status of people from ethnic groups in Britain? *Ethnicity and Health*, 1(5): 33–40.

Aspinall, P.J. and Jacobson, B. (2004) *Ethnic Disparities in Health and Health Care: A Focused Review of the Evidence and Selected Examples of Good Practice*. London: London Health Observatory.

Aspinall, P.J., Jacobson, B. and Polato, G.M. (2003) *Missing Record: The Case for Recording Ethnicity at Birth and Death Registration*. London: London Health Observatory.

Balarajan, R. and Bulusu, L. (1990) Mortality among immigrants in England and Wales 1979–1983, in M. Britton (ed.) *Mortality and Geography: A Review in the Mid-1980s*. London: OPCS.

Blane, D., Power, C. and Bartley, M. (1996) Illness behaviour and the measurement of class differentials in morbidity, *Journal of the Royal Statistical Society*, 156(1): 77–92.

Bracken, P.J., Greenslade, L., Griffin, B. and Smyth, M. (1998) Mental health and ethnicity: an Irish dimension, *British Journal of Psychiatry*, 172: 103–5.

Bradby, H. (1995) Ethnicity: not a black and white issue, a research note, *Sociology of Health and Illness*, 17(3): 405–17.

Bradby, H. (2003) Describing ethnicity in health research, *Ethnicity and Health*, 8(1): 5–13.

Chandola, T. (2001) Ethnic and class differences in health in relation to British South Asians: using the new National Statistics socio-economic classification, *Social Science and Medicine*, 52: 1285–96.

Cochrane, R. and Bal, S.S. (1989) Mental hospital admission rates of immigrants to England: a comparison of 1971 and 1981, *Social Psychiatry and Psychiatric Epidemiology*, 24: 2–11.

DoH (Department of Health) (2001) *Health Survey for England 1999: The Health of Minority Ethnic Groups*. London: The Stationery Office.

DoH (Department of Health) (2005) *Health Survey for England 2004*. London: The Stationery Office.

Erens, B., Primastesta, P. and Prior, G. (eds) (2001) *The Health Survey for England 1999. The Health of Minority Ethnic Groups, Vol 1: Findings. Vol 2: Methodology and Documentation.* London: The Stationery Office.

Feder, G., Crook, A.M., Magee, P., Banerjee, S., Timmis, A.D. and Hemingway, H. (2002) Ethnic differences in management of coronary disease: prospective cohort study of patients undergoing angiography, *British Medical Journal*, 324: 511–16.

Joint Health Surveys Unit of the National Centre for Social Research and University College London (2002) *Ethnic Minority Psychiatric Illness Rates in the Community (EMPIRIC).* London: The Stationery Office.

Karlsen, S. and Nazroo, J.Y. (2002) Relation between racial discrimination, social class and health among ethnic minority groups, *American Journal of Public Health*, 92(4): 624–31.

Knight, T., Smith, Z., Lockton, J., Sahota, P., Bedford, A., Toop, M., Kernohan, E. and Baker, M. (1993) Ethnic differences in risk markers for heart disease in Bradford and implications for preventive strategies, *Journal of Epidemiology and Community Health*, 2: 89–95.

Lear, J.T., Lawrence, I.G., Burden, A.C. and Pohl, J.E.F. (1994) A comparison of stress test referral rates and outcome between Asians and Europeans, *Journal of the Royal Society of Medicine*, 87: 661–2.

Leavey, G. (1999) Suicide and Irish migrants in Britain: identity and integration, *International Review of Psychiatry*, 11(2–3): 168–72.

Maglen, K. (2005) Importing trachoma: the introduction into Britain of American ideas of an 'immigrant disease', 1892–1900, *Immigrants & Minorities*, 23(1): 80–99.

Marmot, M.G., Adelstein, A.M. and Bulusu, L. (1984) *Immigrant Mortality in England and Wales 1970–1978.* London: OPCS HMSO.

Mason, D. (2000) *Race and Ethnicity in Modern Britain*, 2nd edn. Oxford: Oxford University Press.

Modood, T., Berthoud, R., Lakey, J., Nazroo, J., Smith, P., Virdee, S. and Beishon, S. (1997) *Ethnic Minorities in Britain: Diversity and Disadvantage – Fourth National Survey of Ethnic Minorities.* London: Policy Studies Institute.

Nazroo, J. (1997) *The Health of Britain's Ethnic Minorities.* London: Policy Studies Institute.

Nazroo, J.Y. (1998) Genetic, cultural or socio-economic vulnerability? Expanding ethnic inequalities in health, *Sociology of Health and Illness*, 20: 714–34.

Smaje, C. (1995) *Health 'Race' and Ethnicity: Making Sense of the Evidence.* London: The King's Fund.

Sproston, K. and Mindell, J. (2006) *The Health Survey for England 1999, Vol. 1: The Health of Minority Ethnic Groups.* London: The Information Centre.

Tudor-Hart, J. (1971) The inverse care law, *The Lancet*, 27 February: 406–12.

Walls, P. and Williams, R. (2004) Accounting for Irish Catholic ill health in Scotland: a qualitative exploration of some links between 'religion', class and health, *Sociology of Health & Illness*, 26(5): 527.

Wray, H. (2006) The Aliens Act 1905 and the immigration dilemma, *Journal of Law and Society*, 33: 302.

8 Disability and public health: from resistance to empowerment

Nick Watson

Disability and disabled people represent a problem for public health practice. On the one hand, public health must be inclusive, must seek to promote equality and must therefore include disabled people in both its practice and its materials. On the other, public health is about extolling the virtues of health and healthy living while cultural perceptions tend to categorize disabled people as unhealthy or disabled people might acquire their impairment as a consequence of unhealthy lifestyle choices. Public health practitioners therefore have to be both careful and sensitive in planning health promotion activities. Since the prevention of disability is often a stated target of many public health campaigns, from the taking of folic acid in early pregnancy to the reduction of traffic accidents, it can be difficult to avoid the implication that disability is itself a failing.

Counting the number of disabled people in any population is difficult and numbers depend on the definition of disability adopted. It is estimated through data collected by the Disability Follow up to the Family Resources Survey in 1996/7 that in the UK there are about 8.6 million people over 16 who self define as disabled, which is about 15 per cent of the total population (DSS 2000). In 2000 the International Labour Organization (ILO) estimated that there were over 600 million disabled people worldwide with 400 million in low- and middle-income countries (ILO 2000). While the life chances for many disabled people in low- and middle-income countries remain unaltered, it is true to say that the life chances of disabled people in many high-income countries have improved dramatically as a result of social transformation over the last two decades. Much of the drive for these changes has come from the demands of disabled people and their organizations that, through political protests and demonstrations, have sought to redefine disability and disabled people. They have challenged the dominant representation of disability as a medical problem and redefined it as a political or social issue, and have demanded that disability no longer be seen as a personal tragedy. In the UK legislation such as the Disability Discrimination Act, passed in 1995, and the Community Care (Direct Payments) Act of 1996, passed as a direct consequence of the actions of disabled people, has promoted the rights of disabled people to active and full participation in all aspects of life. The discourse that surrounds disability has moved from one of care to one of independence, social participation and civil rights. Mainstream services, such as health and social care organizations have also been criticized for their failure to provide services that meet the needs of disabled people as defined by disabled people themselves, and for reinforcing the idea of disabled people as dependent, frail and vulnerable. An academic study of disability based on a social approach to disability, called disability studies, also emerged as a consequence of this new understanding of disability.

The roots of disability studies emerged as an academic discipline in the mid to late 1970s at roughly the same time as health promotion within public health practice. While modern health promotion theory and practice, it could be argued, owes its origins to the publication of the Lalonde Report in 1974 and the World Health Organization's (WHO) Alma Ata declaration of 1978, so modern disability politics and disability studies emerged as a consequence of the publication of *The Fundamental Principles of Disablement* by the Union of the Physically Impaired Against Segregation (UPIAS) in 1976. These two subject areas might, at first glance, appear to have little in common but they do share some important characteristics; for example they argue for environmental and structural changes to, on the one hand, improve the public health and, on the other, to improve the life chances and opportunities of disabled people. Both represented a rejection of medicine as the solution to the problems they sought to solve and both argued for self-representation and participation in decision making. These two emerging ideas have grown up over the same period yet, despite both engaging with important questions about patterns of power, authority and the human experience, these two fields of study have largely been separate.

The reluctance of disability studies to engage with health promotion theory may in part be a direct consequence of a fear of reinforcing the association between disability and health. Health promotion, despite its many efforts to present an opposite view, is seen by many as being closely linked to medicine and to a medical approach to solving issues associated with the public health. If disability studies were to engage too closely with such a subject area there is a danger that it might be seen as reinforcing links between disability and health. Health promotion's reluctance to engage with disability studies might, on the one hand, be explained by views held by many practitioners that the problems faced by disabled people are medical rather than social and conversely, on the other, a wish to treat disabled people as members of the population and not to single them out as a special group. Whatever the reason, there is very little research exploring health promotion for disabled people. Most research in this area comes from North America and tends, in the main, to treat disability and the problems faced by disabled people and health promotion issues within a medical paradigm. The focus is primarily on the prevention of secondary conditions that an individual with an impairment may be more prone to than a non-disabled person (see for example Rimmer 1999 and Stuifbergen *et al.* 2000).

The social model of disability

In the same way that the Lalonde Report and *Health For All by the Year 2000* set the agenda for health promotion practice and theory so *The Fundamental Principles of Disablement* set the agenda for both disability studies as an academic discipline and disability activism in the UK and internationally. In 1983 Mike Oliver produced what he termed the social model of disability. This was, as he freely acknowledges, based on the UPIAS document and it became the defining characteristic of disability studies and formed the ideological basis of the disabled people's movement. If an article was written within a social model framework it was considered disability studies, if not it was medical sociology. Similarly, if an organization aligned itself with the social model then it was considered part of the progressive movement on disability. Put simply, the social model of disability argues that people are disabled not because of their impairment, but because of the way that society is organized. That is, disability is social in origin. Being disabled by society is about discrimination that restricts individuals with impairments and any link between disability and impairment is rejected. The model is based on the two seminal definitions of impairment and disability. Impairment is lacking all or part of a limb, or having a defective limb, organism or mechanism of the body while disability is the disadvantage or restriction of activity caused by a contemporary social organization that takes no or little account of people who have physical impairments and thus excludes them from the mainstream of social activities (UPIAS 1976: 3–4).

This is a structural analysis, based on the notion of disabled people as an oppressed minority group, and disablement as a collective experience. Disability is viewed as a problem located within society and the way to reduce disability is to alter the social and physical environment. The removal of social barriers to the reintegration of people with physical impairments eliminates disability itself (Finkelstein 1980: 33).

The social model of disability mirrors early second wave feminists. Where feminists distinguished sex and gender, the former physical and the latter social and cultural (Oakley 1972) so the social model separates disablement and impairment. Much of the research in disability studies focuses on the disabling environment, that is the physical and social barriers that exclude disabled people and render them powerless and voiceless.

The social model is not without its critics. Attention has for example been drawn to the less than effective manner with which the social model reconciles dimensions of gender (Morris 1999), race and ethnicity (Vernon 1996), class (Williams 1983), generation (Shakespeare and Watson 1997) identity and sexuality (Shakespeare *et al.* 1996), and impairment (Hughes and Patterson 1997; Shakespeare and Watson 2001) within or alongside disability. However, as Oliver (2004) has recently argued, the social model provides a useful tool both as a guide for providing services to disabled people and as a means to evaluate how services are delivered to disabled people.

Disability as an inequality issue

The available research presents overwhelming evidence that discrimination against disabled people is widespread. Colin Barnes's study (1990) was perhaps the first to provide the most complete evidence for such discrimination. This study documents the inequality experienced by disabled people in a wide range of social arenas including those of education, work, healthcare, housing, social care, leisure and politics. Other work, such as that of Hyde (1996) on employment, the Thomas (1997) research on parenthood, the Barton (1995) study on education, and that of Zarb and Oliver (1993) on ageing, just adds weight to these claims. Clearly disabled people can be represented as an oppressed group and the discrimination they experience cuts across a number of different policy arenas including social care, healthcare, employment, education, housing and transport (for discussion of attempts to link policy across these areas see Chapters 11, 12, 13 and 14).

There is also compelling evidence to suggest that disabled people are subject to inequalities in health. A recent report by the Disability Rights Commission, *Equal Treatment: Closing the Gap*, clearly documents these inequalities and the Commission has identified the reduction of health inequalities between disabled and non disabled people as one of its ten priority areas (DRC 2006). This report shows, for example, how people with an enduring mental health problem are more than twice as likely as other people to have diabetes, are more likely to have heart disease, stroke or hypertension and are 60 per cent more likely to smoke. Other research has shown how people with a visual impairment are more likely to die of cancer than their non disabled peers (Beverley *et al.* 2002). Disabled people are also more likely to exhibit lifestyle risk factors associated with poor health. For example, people with a learning difficulty are more likely to be obese and less likely to eat a healthy diet (Robertson *et al.* 2000). People with other impairments also have a tendency to obesity. Disabled people are less likely to be physically active and take part in sport; they also face discrimination in access to primary care services. (Morris 1999). Disabled people also face discrimination in access to healthcare, either at a primary care level or at secondary care (ODPM 2005).

Despite the evidence of such widespread health inequalities there is little written within the inequalities literature to suggest that disability is seen as a cause of health inequalities. It is recognized that poverty has a strong interrelationship with disability, with the World Bank estimating that over 20 per cent of disability is the result of poverty, and disability is often seen as a marker of social inequality, in that people from lower socioeconomic groupings are more likely to report a long standing illness, disability or mental health problem and also in that the onset of disability can exacerbate pre-existing disadvantage (Acheson 1998). Disability is not seen in the same way as, for example, social class, ethnicity or gender.

If it is accepted that one of the underlying principles of health promotion is the tackling of inequalities both within and between nations then surely health promotion should be seeking to address such inequalities. The recently published policy document *Improving the Life Chances of Disabled People* makes it clear that wider efforts to address and reduce health inequalities would be undermined by a failure to reduce disability inequality (ODPM 2005).

Public health and disability

If, as has been argued, disabled people face widespread social and economic exclusion, as well as inequalities in health, what should the focus of public health for disabled people be? The focus could be on helping disabled people challenge discrimination, stigma or social exclusion, promoting their right to full participation in society. Alternatively it could concentrate on providing disabled people with information and advice on health-related matters such as smoking, diet and exercise as well as more directed advice on living with their impairment. The chosen strategy, of course, depends on public perceptions of the nature of public health, although it would appear that much UK national policy would favour the latter. Recent policy directives from, for example, Health Challenge Wales, Health Scotland and NICE all point to a focus on behaviour change with little emphasis on what Tones and Tilford (2001) would term radical health promotion. While it is obviously important that public health practitioners challenge risk factors such as smoking, diet and exercise there is also a need to tackle the social and political conditions that contribute to people's ill health. There is certainly widespread evidence to suggest that disabled people adopt more unhealthy lifestyles compared to non disabled people, as highlighted above. However, for many disabled people smoking, a lack of exercise or other health behaviour may be only a trivial concern in their day-to-day struggle. If public health is to be of use to disabled people then it must tackle the causes of disablement. It needs to direct its main efforts at the causes of the oppression that disabled people face rather than the symptoms (for the effectiveness of integrated policy on health including upstream approaches, see in particular Chapter 11).

There is however little evidence to suggest that public health currently offers much for disabled people or seeks to include them, with much evidence suggesting that they are currently excluded from public health practice. Work by Burns and Cohen (1998) for example documents how people with a severe mental health problem receive significantly less health promotion through general practitioners compared to those without a mental health problem. This is despite the fact that consultation rates are significantly higher than for people without mental health problems. The same is true of people with a learning difficulty, who research suggests are far less likely to receive health checks, be part of well women groups or other health needs assessment (Broughton and Thompson 2000). The Disability Rights Commission's investigation into the inequalities in health experienced by people with a mental health problem or learning difficulty supports these findings (DRC 2006). American research suggests that adults with a mobility impairment are less likely to receive blood pressure checks, have their blood cholesterol screened or receive other health advice than their non disabled peers (Coyle *et al.* 2000). What little activity there is tends in the main to focus either on behaviour change or symptom management. This latter approach forms the basis of what is termed *The Expert Patient* (DoH 2002), a major theme in current health policy in the UK.

The Expert Patient programme is based on ideas developed at the Stanford Patient Education Research Center (Lorig *et al.* 2006). This approach suggests that disabled people can best be helped by encouraging self management, by which individuals are taught to live with their condition and given the confidence to deal with health service professionals. They are also instructed about role management and the emotional management of their condition. The initiative aims to move patients from being passive recipients of care to agents actively involved in the self management of their care. It aims to empower participants to take responsibility for the management of their condition and to work in partnership with health and social care professionals and so take greater control over their lives. It is a highly structured, standardized programme with a strong element of patient education. The course content includes sections on disease related problem solving, managing emotions, exercise, relaxation, nutrition and communication skills, as well as advice on managing medications and using the healthcare system. It is very much a top down approach.

The idea of empowering people to take control of their own health is a distinctive feature of health promotion as enshrined in the Ottawa Charter (WHO 1986). In that sense the Expert Patient programme is an enablement strategy through which it is hoped people with a chronic condition or other impairment can achieve their fullest health potential. However, its focus on problems associated with an individual's impairment and its failure to examine wider social determinants of health, such as access to work, to education, to housing or to other areas of life such as the provision of personal assistance or direct payments which may be important to disabled people would suggest that rather than enabling and empowering disabled people, the Expert Patient programme, through its focus on the medical, runs the risk of disempowering them.

The medicalization of disability through health promotion is also found in other strategies. For example, work on the promotion of exercise for people with a severe mental health problem, including schizophrenia and hallucinations, suggests that exercise can act as an adjunct to treatment (Faulkner and Biddle 1999). Other health benefits are ignored. It may well be argued that this approach merely reflects the needs of people with a mental health problem or other impairment and that generic health promotion is not a priority. There is some evidence to suggest that disabled people might benefit from targeted health promotion or wellness programmes that are developed specifically to meet their needs. It has been reported that many disabled people have what are described as secondary conditions (Seekins *et al.* 1994; Coyle *et al.* 2000). These included fatigue, obesity, lack of physical fitness, spasticity and joint pain, some of which may be amenable to tertiary health prevention interventions. It is suggested that if people were to be given advice on how to avoid these conditions then their quality of life would improve. It could be argued that such an analysis ignores the evidence around inequalities in health and everyday life experienced by disabled people. Indeed, in both studies above the respondents cited lack of access, such as to buildings and toilets, as a major factor that affected their quality of life.

The social model leads practitioners to suggest that public health for disabled people is about tackling and removing barriers such as these. There is strong empirical evidence to support the view that the removal of such barriers does improve the health of disabled people. Work by Barlow and Venables (2004) and Dewsbury *et al.* (2004) shows how the design of appropriate housing and technological aids has the potential to enable older and disabled people to maintain quality of life. Research by Haywood (2001) documents how nearly 75 per cent of disabled people claim that their health has improved as a direct result of housing adaptations. The link between unemployment and poor mental and physical wellbeing is well established. The Disability Rights Commission estimates that only 51 per cent of disabled people are in work, falling to 21 per cent of people with a mental health condition and 17 per cent of people with a learning disability. This is an important target area of public health for disabled people. The wellbeing of disabled people, as is the case with non disabled people, is better preserved when they live their lives as active members of a healthy community (for discussion of the research evidence linking participation, communities and health see Chapter 6; for an assessment of the success of initiatives towards building healthy communities see Chapters 11, 12, 13, 14 and 16). The development and maintenance of healthy communities is a stated aim of many public health initiatives and is enshrined in documents such as the Ottawa Charter, which seeks to promote active participating communities. It would be reasonable to expect progress towards a safe and secure environment with good social support. However, evidence suggests that while such programmes are now fairly well widespread throughout the UK, there is little involvement of disabled people in these activities (Edwards 2001).

Public health for disabled people is an area that is currently underdeveloped. While there are programmes of work that include disabled people there is little evidence of work that is both aimed specifically at disabled people and also focused on social barriers rather than on individual impairments. This preoccupation with impairment can reinforce the whole concept of individualization of disability, encouraging disabled people to run their lives around the management of symptoms rather than tackle the causes. It may well be argued that health promotion practitioners have little expertise in this latter area and, as a consequence, are better placed to focus on the former (for an assessment of the efficacy of approaches base on advocacy, see Chapter 11). If this is the case then public health policy would improve with a focus on how health promotion packages can best be designed to meet the individual needs of disabled people and on whether disabled people are better served by inclusion within mainstream programmes or whether there is a need to design specific courses and materials.

In part, these problems can be solved with research on the sources and practices that underpin the generation of knowledge about public health for disabled people. There is both a need and a demand for some individual health promotion focusing on, for example, smoking, diet or exercise. There is also a recognized need to develop activities that aim to increase individual understanding of impairment, the health service and other issues associated with self management (Lorig *et al.* 2006). However, such approaches need to be augmented with an element that explores wider social issues. How great an element and in what particular areas can be resolved only by working with disabled people. This might, in part, be helped by the use of disability equality training. This is a concept developed by organizations of disabled people (Gillespie-Sells and Campbell 1991). It aims to focus on disability rather than impairment and challenges understandings of disability, promoting a social rather than individual model of disability. Crucially it involves disabled people in its design and delivery. It is only through engagement with disabled people that public health can develop a model that will allow for a dynamic approach; one that recognizes difference and respects individual need, while at the same time challenging the social barriers that serve to exclude disabled people.

References

Acheson, D. (1998) *Independent Inquiry into Inequalities in Health.* London: The Stationery Office.

Barlow, J. and Venables, T. (2004) Will technological innovation create the lifetime home? *Housing Studies*, 19(5): 795–810.

Barnes, C. (1990) *Disabled People in Britain: The Case for Anti-discrimination Legislation.* London: Falmer Press.

Beverley, C., Bath, P. and Booth, A. (2002) *The Health Information Needs of Visually Impaired Groups.* Final report for the National Assembly of Wales. Cardiff: National Assembly of Wales.

Broughton, S. and Thomson, K. (2000) Women with learning disabilities: risk behaviours and experiences of the cervical smear, *Journal of Advanced Nursing*, 32(4): 905–12.

Burns, T. and Cohen, A. (1998) Item of service payments for general practitioner care of severely mentally ill patients: does the money matter? *British Journal of General Practice*, 48: 1415–16.

Coyle, C.P., Santiago, M.C., Shank, J.W., Ma, G.X. and Boyd, R. (2000) Secondary conditions and women with physical disabilities: a descriptive study, *Archives of Physical Medicine and Rehabilitation*, 81: 1380–7.

Dewsbury, G., Rouncefield, M., Clarke, K. and Sommerville, I. (2004) Depending on digital design: ending exclusivity, *Housing Studies*, 19(5): 811–25.

DoH (Department of Health) (2002) *The Expert Patient: A New Approach to Chronic Disease Management in the 21st Century*. London: DoH.

DRC (Disability Rights Commission) (2006) *Equal Treatment: Closing the Gap*. Interim report of a formal investigation into health inequalities, www.drc-gb.org/newsroom/health investigation.asp (accessed 10 April 2006).

DSS (Department of Social Security) (2000) *Disability Follow-up to the 1996/97 Family Resources Survey*. SN: 4090. Colchester: Data Archive.

Edwards, C. (2001) Inclusion in regeneration: a place for disabled people? *Urban Studies*, 38(2): 267–86.

Faulkner, G. and Biddle, S. (1999) Exercise as an adjunct treatment for schizophrenia: a review of the literature, *Journal of Mental Health*, 8(5): 441–57.

Finkelstein, V. (1980) *Attitudes and Disabled People*. New York: World Rehabilitation Fund.

Gillespie-Sells, K. and Campbell, J. (1991) *Disability Equality Training Trainers Guide*. London: CCETSW.

Haywood, E. (2001) *Money Well Spent: The Effectiveness and Value of Housing Adaptations*. London: Policy Press.

Hughes, B. and Patterson, K. (1997) The social model of disability and the disappearing body: towards a sociology of impairment, *Disability and Society*, 12(3): 325–40.

Hyde, M. (1996) Fifty years of failure: employment services for disabled people in the UK, *Work, Employment and Society*, 10: 683–700.

ILO (International Labour Organization) (2000) *Unlocking the Evidence*. Employers' forum on disability. Geneva: ILO.

Lalonde, M. (1974) *A New Perspective on the Health of Canadians*. Ottawa: Government of Canada.

Lorig, K., Holman, H., Sobel, D., Lauren, D., González, V. and Minor, M. (2006) *Living a Healthy Life with Chronic Conditions: Self-Management of Heart Disease, Arthritis, Stroke, Diabetes, Asthma, Bronchitis, Emphysema and Others,* 3rd edn. Boulder, CO: Bull Publishing.

Morris, J. (1999) *Hurtling into a Void: Transition to Adulthood for Young Disabled People with 'Complex Health and Support Needs'*. Brighton: Pavilion Publishing.

Oakley, A. (1972) *Sex, Gender and Society*. London: M. Temple Smith.

Oliver, M. (2004) If I had a hammer: the social model in action, in C. Barnes (ed.) *The Social Model of Disability: Theory and Research*. Leeds: The Disability Press.

ODPM (2005) *Improving the Life Chances of Disabled People*. London: Office of the Deputy Prime Minister.

Rimmer, M. (1999) Health promotion for people with disabilities: the emerging paradigm shift from disability prevention to prevention of secondary conditions, *Physical Therapy*, 79(5): 495–502.

Robertson, J., Emerson, E., Gregory, N., Hatton, C., Turner, S., Kessissoglou, S. and Hallam, A. (2000) Lifestyle related risk factors for poor health in residential settings for people with intellectual disabilities, *Research in Developmental Disabilities*, 21: 469–86.

Seekins, T., Clay, J. and Ravesloot, C. (1994) A descriptive study of secondary conditions reported by a population of adults with physical disabilities served by three independent living centers in a rural state, *Journal of Rehabilitation*, 60: 47–51.

Shakespeare, T. and Watson, N. (1997) Defending the social model, *Disability and Society*, 12(2): 293–300.

Shakespeare, T. and Watson, N. (2001) The social model of disability: an outdated ideology? *Exploring Theories and Expanding Methodologies*, 2: 9–28.

Shakespeare, T., Gillespie-Sells, K. and Davies, D. (1996) *Untold Desires: The Sexual Politics of Disability*. London: Cassell.

Stuifbergen, A.K., Seraphine, A. and Roberts, G. (2000) An explanatory model of health promotion and quality of life in chronic disabling conditions, *Nursing Research*, 49(3): 122–9.

Thomas, C. (1997) The baby and the bathwater: disabled people and motherhood in social context, *Sociology of Health and Illness*, 19: 622–43.

Tones, K. and Tilford, S. (2001) *Health Promotion: Effectiveness, Efficiency and Equity*. Cheltenham: Nelson Thornes.

UPIAS (1976) *The Fundamental Principles of Disablement*. London: UPIAS.

Vernon, A. (1996) A stranger in many camps: the experience of disabled black and ethnic minority women, in J. Morris (ed.) *Encounters with Strangers: Feminism and Disability*. London: Women's Press.

WHO (1978) Primary health care: Report of the international conference on primary health care, Alma-Ata, USSR, 6-12 September 1978 Geneva: World Health Organisation.

WHO (1986) *The Ottawa Charter for Health Promotion: An International Conference of Health Promotion*. Copenhagen: WHO.

Williams, G. (1983) The movement for independent living: an evaluation and critique, *Social Science and Medicine*, 17(15): 1003–10.

Zarb, G. and Oliver, M. (1993) *Ageing with a disability: What Do they Expect after all these Years?* London: University of Greenwich.

9 Mass media, lifestyle and public health

Martin King

The recognition of health and the media as a discrete area for academic study is a relatively new phenomenon (Seale 2003; King and Watson 2005) with the assertion that an audience's perception of health issues and health policy is, at least partly, shaped by its presentation in the media. This has come about as educators and researchers have recognized the value of using techniques associated with media and cultural studies to interrogate the increasing number of health texts available for public consumption (King and Watson 2001). These include television, film, print media and the internet, as well as the more traditional public health campaign materials used by practitioners.

This area of study has drawn together a number of works relating to health and lifestyle in the media including health, lifestyle and consumption (Featherstone 1991; Baudrillard 1998), medico morality (Petersen 1994; Lyons and Willott 1999), theories of individualization (Bauman 2001), behaviour regulation (Lupton 2003) and audience reception of public health campaigns (Southwell 2000; Doi 2005).

Health on television

The role of the mass media in modern society is well documented elsewhere. This chapter focuses on health on television with particular reference to the recent phenomenon of public health television as an emergent branch of lifestyle television that has grown in popularity since the mid 1990s. While examples of this exist in other media, such as the film *Supersize Me* (2004) or the plethora of lifestyle magazines particularly aimed at young women, television has grown to be the key, perhaps most intrusive, medium in modern society.

Within the UK there are a number of health-related television genres with a long history. Hospital-based dramas, such as *Casualty* and *Holby City*, remain as popular as ever while the imported American *ER* has led to a number of offspring. Hospital-based comedy too has been very popular since the *Carry on* and *Doctor* films which began in the late 1950s. Contemporary offerings in the UK of this tradition include *No Angels* and the increasingly surreal *Green Wing*.

Health television in the early twenty first century, however, offers a reconceptualization of health as a reflection of challenges to the medical model (O'Brien, 1995) promoted by a number of authors in the public health field (seminal contributors include Lalonde 1974; Naidoo and Wills 1994; Seedhouse 1997, 2003). O'Brien (1995) suggests the blurring of health and lifestyle is a dangerous development, a dedifferentiation of health and social life (for a comparable perception, see Bunton *et al.* 1995). The complaint that health has been colonized in the name of lifestyle (O'Brien 1995: 203) is underlined by television programme makers' interest in this area in the last decade. The danger of this approach being linked to individual responsibility for health was recognized by Davison *et al.* (1997: 75), who identified the new interest in lifestyle as an officially sponsored ideological perspective with its emphasis on personal responsibility for the maintenance of health and the avoidance of chronic disease. This is in marked contrast to the intentions of authors like Seedhouse (1997) who sought to create models of health which included structural as well as individual solutions to health inequalities and the major contemporary causes of death and disability (for further discussion of models of health, both individual and structural, see Chapter 4; for discussion of lifestyle in the context of public health see Chapter 11).

This ideological shift can be seen in UK party politics with New Labour's approach to improving public health. The focus on individual responsibility for health in Labour's *Prevention and Health: Everybody's Business* (DoH 1976) is revisited in New Labour's *Saving Lives* (DoH 1999) and the project continues in *Choosing Health* (DoH 2004), where the idea that communities and public/private-sector organizations may also be influential in improving the public health seems to have been abandoned. Indeed, there is a return to a spirit of individualism, an approach that seems remarkably similar to that contained in the Conservative government's *The Health of the Nation* (DoH 1992) (for overviews of the history and success of public health intervention see Chapter 2 and Chapter 11).

Morality and health

The connections made between health, disease aetiology, morality and responsibility have ancient cultural roots (Brandt and Rozin 1997). There are a number of texts which explore the way that media coverage of health issues is underpinned by discourses of judgementalism and morality – for example, Courtwright (1997) on drug use and Gordon (1997) on teenage pregnancy.

The rise of lifestyle television can be viewed within this context, where individual lifestyle change leads to health improvement and increasingly the emphasis is on self-discipline and illness is interpreted as a failure to regulate the self (Petersen 1994). Leichter (1997) has coined the term 'lifestyle correctness' to describe this phenomenon as part of the new wellness movement. With both government policy and lifestyle television focusing on longer, fulfilling, healthier lives, he points to an identifiable subtext of social status. Mirroring ideas put forward by Baudrillard (1998), Leichter claims that by defining acceptable and unacceptable lifestyles, poorer sections of society are increasingly marginalized since the maintenance of a healthy lifestyle also encourages mass consumption. King and Watson (2005) describe this process as a distancing of the well wealthies from the poorly poors and argue that morality discourses underpin health and lifestyle programming (for further discussion of increasing inequality and its consequences, see Chapter 4).

Moreover, a complex health matrix is inscribed in the look better, feel better obsession with lifestyle simulations in contemporary western societies. The media utilize therapeutic discourse, often of a moralistic kind, as a way of framing the action on the screen. Lives are potentially transformed from unhealthy/chaotic to healthy/orderly and in the process the viewer is encouraged to see the potential transformation: towards living morally, if not actually, healthier lives. Within the UK examples of this before and after narrative of programmes include *Home Front* and *Changing Rooms*. John Ellis (1999), for example, has argued that television is a form of therapy where viewers are helped to work through the problems and chaos of their lives. According to Gripsrud (2002) this is the illusion of transformation, a televisual and temporally boundaried promise that for this time, in this space, viewers can experience emotions of change reminiscent of the Seedhouse foundations model of health (Seedhouse 1997) with its ideas about individuals effecting change and moving towards better health. The increasingly popular chat shows, such as the imported *Oprah, Jenny* and *Ricki* (Shattuc 1997) or the home-grown *Jeremy Kyle* and *Trisha* provide prime examples of these morality discourses in action.

It has been suggested that this surge in popularity of lifestyle programming is in response to a need of postmodern societies to simulate order and that this need has been combined with powerful and often moralistic discourses of order, cleanliness and anti-infection characteristic of western societies. Additional stimulus in this direction has been as a response to globalization and the perceived threat of global contamination and disorder made partially visible through the very same media (Brandt and Rozin 1997; King and Watson 2005). (For further discussion of globalization, boundaries and disease, see Chapters 3 and 10).

The roots of these ideas, however, can be traced back to the European Enlightenment in the eighteenth century, while notions of moral and economic self-determination were combined with the privatization of family and home in the nineteenth century. These and the emergence of the concept of suburbs, the separation of work from home life and the institutionalization of differential gender roles all provided the groundwork for the emergence of magazines such as *Good Housekeeping* (Bunton 1997) and subsequently of a lifestyle discourse. Dirt and disorder has been a recurring motif of public health (Pryce 2005) and is now manifest in the healthy lifestyle programming, a contemporary version of 'now wash your hands' notices.

An interesting development has been the emergence of a discourse of shame, where victims are blamed for their poor taste in dress (*What Not to Wear*), untidy homes (*How Clean is your House?*) or lack of parenting skills (*Honey, We're Killing the Kids*). In these programmes, a negation of the abject allows for the mainstreaming of bourgeois respectability. It can be seen then that the mass media itself has the potential to create particular conversations through subtle reinforcement of healthy notions of living but which are themselves informed by the cultural prerequisites of a political order.

Public health and the mass media

It is often suggested that public health campaigns have little effect on behaviour (Baggaley 1991). Influential public health initiatives such as the Stanford Three Community Project (Davis 1987) and theonly Finnish North Karelia Project (Koselka *et al.* 1976) have been combined with studies from advertising and academic authors emerging from the new public health movement (see Tones 1985; Lefebvre 1992; Wallack *et al.* 1993) to produce a body of knowledge focused on the strengths and limitations of the use of the media in public health (for further work on the effectiveness of public health, see Chapter 11; for an overview of mass media interventions for public health, see Hubley 2005).

Public health practitioners and policy makers have often failed to draw on this knowledge when planning new initiatives. For example, an examination of the content of public information films in their changing political context, between the late 1950s and early 1980s, reveals interesting attempts to reconceptualize public health at various stages in the late twentieth century and to rewrite health messages accordingly (King 2003). Lessons about the difference between using the media for awareness raising and behaviour change also emerge. Keith Tones's work on this subject still remains the benchmark (Tones 1985; Tones *et al.* 1994).

Public health television

Public health television is the broadcasting of public health issues that become information and entertainment. This is a relatively new development of lifestyle television over the past two years and can be identified in a number of ways. First, older lifestyle transformation programmes in the UK, such as Trinny and Susannah's *What Not to Wear*, emphasize the health benefits of lifestyle change. For example, the last series of Trinny and Susannah shifted the emphasis from not only looking better to also feeling better; boosting self-confidence by linking outer and inner change. Second, the primetime viewing slots and the associated audience viewing figures given to these programmes indicate the creation of a new genre by programmers.

A good example of this is *Are You Younger Than You Think*. Broadcast in a primetime Saturday-night slot on the UK's BBC1 in July 2005 and hosted by the popular sports presenter Des Lynam, it used a mixture of quiz format, celebrity guests and regional link-ups to examine lifestyle and its relationship to the body and ageing as a sort of Baudrillard for the masses. As the title indicates, *Honey, We're Killing the Kids* is a good old-fashioned shock horror health education approach (see for example Maibach and Parrott 1995) where parents, aided by computer imaging, are allowed to see what the results of their poor lifestyle choices will be on their offspring when they reach 40. In 2005 this programme moved from the minority channel BBC3 to BBC1 because of its success.

Even more popular was *Jamie's School Dinners*, in which, week by week, chef Jamie Oliver utilized a contemporary obsession with celebrity to draw attention to the appalling state of school meals in the UK. The public press outcry and popular attention in which viewing figures peaked at 5 million, a very large audience for Channel 4, pressured the government towards action, something public health practitioners have been trying to do via traditional health education, local initiatives and the development of healthy schools awards and local policy developments for 20 years. In May 2006 Education Secretary Alan Johnson announced new nutritional standards for school meals and the banning of junk food (www.news.bbc.co.uk, 2006). This has to be recognized as an example of the power of public health television. It also illustrates Leichter's (1997) arguments about lifestyle correctness and the gap between the poorly poors and the wealthy wells. Jamie's most hated item on the school dinner menu, the turkey twizzler, was much loved by children on the programme and sales subsequently rose, while low-paid school meals staff were expected to prepare and cook fresh meals in the time previously allocated for opening and heating up frozen foodstuffs (www.news.bbc.co.uk 2005).

The third feature of public health television is its recognition of contemporary public health issues as identified by government. Food, fat and smoking become key targets with solutions identified as the responsibility of individuals. This interconnection of ideas will be explored further in case studies.

Lonsdale (2006) examines this new phenomenon and raises questions about the role of such programming in ongoing public health initiatives. The fact that these programmes have proved popular with viewers has provided a motivation for television companies to produce more. Lisa Ausden, BBC Executive Producer on *Fat Nation* and *Diet Trial,* draws attention to obesity as the both the most significant contemporary health issue and one with which people should be engaged (Lonsdale 2006: 14).

Ausden attributes *Fat Nation's* lack of popularity in comparison to Channel 4's *You Are What You Eat* to its lower-key approach. *You Are What You Eat* featured overweight participants laying out all the food they ate in a week on a table, and on-screen colonic irrigation, raising questions about whether it is a creative approach to education on obesity or merely spectacle or car crash television (Lonsdale 2006). Parallels can be drawn with Jane Shattuc's (1997) work on the claims of television talk shows such as *The Ricki Lake Show* and *The Jerry Springer Show* to be part of a populist approach to the 'talking cure'. In *You Are What You Eat,* Dr Gillian McKeith draws on the discourse of scientific research to justify her methods. Similarly, the BBC's *Diet Trials* was a collaboration with the University of Surrey and claimed to be a scientific weight loss experiment (Lonsdale 2006).

Is, then, the use of the public health agenda by television producers and programmers a positive or negative development for the advancement of the cause of public health? Has public health as entertainment resulted in public health benefit? Using three short case studies these questions will be examined further.

Case studies

The three case studies chosen all date from early 2006 and are an illustration of the type of public health television programming discussed previously.

Documentary research is a useful way of examining society through texts produced in that society at a particular time (May 1997). Texts can be seen as products of the social, political and ideological context in which they were produced. The use of case studies in this type of research is well established (Stake 1998). The work here draws on the work of van Dijk (1993) and Fairclough (1995) and utilizes a framework of textual analysis within discourse analysis. It examines issues of production and reception in texts, including the examination of settings, roles and positions of the actors in the text, genre, signs and speech acts. McKee (2003) refers to this process as poststructural textual analysis.

The analysis will draw on some of the ideas discussed earlier in the chapter and will explore some of the issues raised by this new phenomenon.

Cold Turkey

Cold Turkey is an hour-long one-off production in the UK in which two bad-girl celebrities, Tara Palmer-Tomkinson and Sophie Anderton, both with tabloid newspaper and populist television credentials, attempt to give up their last addiction of smoking. Framed, then, by two public health credos of New Labour, smoking and passive smoking, the programme focuses on individual responsibility and the battle of giving up. Seale (2003) has looked exclusively at the use of war-based metaphors in the media with particular reference to cancer and this programme has them in abundance.

The two celebrities featured are famed for previous battles won against other addictions, Palmer-Tomkinson with cocaine and Anderton with alcohol. The programme, therefore, sets up a new challenge for these seasoned campaigners and opens with them defiantly posing before the camera. There is a titillating aura to the introduction based upon the audience knowledge of stories associated with them including their appearance and demeanour, and the phallic symbolism of the cigarettes they are holding. This observation supports producer Lisa Ausden's comments about the visual treatment of the subject being important to draw the audience in (Lonsdale 2006).

This introduction is contrasted with the environment of their encounter with the stop smoking specialist from the Tobacco Addiction Unit at a famous London teaching hospital, St Bartholomew's. The setting, which is white, clinical and hospital like, adds gravitas, as does the doctor in his white coat.

The programme revolves on this juxtaposition, adding a sexual component to a recognizable health education approach to smoking cessation. The viewers are given information about smoking-related deaths by the specialist, who then uses aversion therapy to encourage the participants to quit. Using conventional shock tactics (Maibach and Parrott 1995) it can be seen as a sort of twenty first-century version of the diseased lung in a jar.

The hour explores the personal and individual accounts of the two participants, drawing on discourses of morality and individual responsibility. There is a bad and badder theme with the determined Sophie pitted against the spoilt, petulant and cheating Tara, who claims to have given up for several days, but is caught out in the end. The programme draws on the conflicting character narratives popular in other UK television formats, such as *Big Brother* and *I'm A Celebrity*. The producers, therefore, introduce the public health issue within formats understood by and familiar to audiences. The conclusion reflects the spirit of the politics of New Labour's *Choosing Health* (DoH 2004): one fails, one succeeds and it is up to the individual to find a way.

Superslim Me

While *Cold Turkey* adopts a serious approach to its subject matter, indicated by the association of the title with heroin addiction and its choice of previously addicted celebrities, *Superslim Me* takes, by its own admission, a fun look at losing weight. It draws together a number of interesting media components and applies them to a public health topic. Like *Celebrity Fit Club* and its associated products, it is both a serious attempt to address a key public health issue and a voyeuristic spectacle. Lorraine Kelly, with her reputation on UK daytime television for homely friendliness and common sense, is the host. As Geertz (1983: 84) notes, 'as a frame of thought ... common sense is as totalizing as any other, no religion is more dogmatic, no science more ambitious, no philosophy more general' in its claims to reach things as they are. Lorraine draws on this common-sense frame of thought to the full in identifying herself with the audience. This ability has been the cornerstone of her career and defines a context for what follows.

The premise of the programme is that ten women weighing more than 13 stone will each try a popular diet for a period of two weeks. The short-term concern of public health television is brought into sharp focus by the task. Present is an obesity specialist and Tania, a slim dietician without a surname whose physical attributes are designed to contrast with the participants following a format familiar to audiences from such programmes as *What Not to Wear*. The tone of the programme indicates fun. The women each tackle diets including the Cambridge, the Atkins, the F-Plan and the Macrobiotic. A hint of experiment and scientific medicine, with medical checks and weigh-ins, is juxtaposed against games playing and competition. The programme ends with a rundown of the top ten in order of weight loss.

For the participants weight has serious health implications. Moreover, although the issue of media pressure is tackled at the outset with celebrities discussing the whole notion of the perfect body, they do so against juxtaposed tabloid magazine headlines such as 'You Fat Bitch' and a hostess who ensures that expectations of fun and common sense predominate.

Following a section on the F-Plan diet there is a jokey discussion about high fibre in which lavatorial humour abounds. The crankiness of the macrobiotic diet is contrasted with more sensible approaches, again drawing on the concept of lifestyle correctness (Leichter 1997) and common sense. Any serious attempts to address public health issues seem to be undermined by the final words of the hostess where she confesses that, for her, diets are entirely counterproductive. However, the fact that the programme attempted to raise awareness about the nature and content of a number of popular diets could be read as of health interest even if a two-week attempt at behaviour change can be dismissed as short-term spectacle.

The Carole Caplin Treatment

This series comprised a number of half-hour shows in a late afternoon slot on UK television's Channel 4. The celebrity status of the hostess, Carole Caplin, results from her role as the lifestyle adviser to Cherie Blair, the wife of the British Prime Minister. The setting and surroundings for this show are vital in creating a set of associations with alternative therapy and holistic lifestyle. Hall draws on the work of the French structuralist philosopher Michel Foucault to explain the way in which representation in the media works through language as 'any signifying system' of signs (Hall 1997: 6).

In the opening sequence the viewer sees the hostess dressed in white, surrounded by cream furnishings, glass tables, candles, flowers and burning incense. An impression of tranquillity suggests to the audience the idea of the guru at home.

Drawing in a number of alternative therapists and presided over by Carole, the format of the show is that of the transformation of two subjects. The presenter takes care at the beginning to ground herself in the common-sense world made familiar by the previous case. The assumptions of the transformations that follow include those of contemporary public health documents like *Choosing Health* (DoH 2004) and those of the body project of Baudrillard (1998). At one point one of the participants even says that she is under construction. The subjects appear to be chosen to represent a particular grouping or even a stereotype (Hall 1997). Sharon, a Manchester cancer-surviving single mother who wants to take a journey back to good health is juxtaposed with Naomi, a high achiever, exercise enthusiast who wants to lose weight and reduce her stress levels.

The holistic approach offered draws on ideas advanced by authors like Seedhouse (1997) and critiques of the biomedical approach (McKeown 1976). The programme can be read as an exercise in awareness-raising about the value of alternative therapies to deal with individual health issues. It is very much rooted in the idea of individual responsibility and self-help promotion (Brandt and Rozin 1997). The personal narrative format is similar to that shared by Tara and Sophie in their attempts to give up smoking, but what is provided in all three shows are ideas and exposure to methods people may not have thought of, in formats which are familiar to them.

Public health television: education or indoctrination?

The question for public health practitioners is whether such programmes as described here have a legitimate awareness raising role. The critique offered here has focused on the political and ideological context. Such media interest in public health television may also be short-lived. Lonsdale (2006) reports that the BBC's programme schedule for 2006 contained lower levels of such programming than in the previous year. BBC producer Lisa Ausden is also sceptical of the public health value beyond entertainment since the obesity crisis in the UK is building despite saturation programming about weight problems (Lonsdale 2006: 15).

This would suggest that programme makers themselves are less concerned about outcomes than ratings. Add to that concerns around misinformation, indoctrination, ethics and morality and it would be reasonable to conclude that the development is not beneficial in public health terms.

On the other hand, the public health agenda has been wrested away from professionals and practitioners into the light of primetime television slots and that is an interesting development. Lonsdale (2006) argues that reinvention around subject matter and a search for novelty in presentation provides a stark contrast to the tiresome didactic message approach often associated with public health campaigns. And given the chequered history of the relationship between public health and the mass media (King 2003) the popularity of public health television could be seen as a willingness of the public to engage with a range of public health issues, which could be a useful starting point for practitioners.

References

Anonymous (2005) *Cash Concerns over School Meals*, www.news.bbc.co.uk, accessed 19 May 2006.

Anonymous (2006) *Junk Food banned in Schools*, www.news.bbc.co.uk, accessed 19 May 2006.

Baggaley, J. (1991) Media health Campaigns: not just what you say but the way you say it, in WHO, *AIDS Prevention through Health Promotion: Facing Sensitive Issues*. Amsterdam: WHO.

Baudrillard, J. (1998) *The Consumer Society: Myths and Structures*. London: Sage.

Bauman, Z. (2001) *The Individualised Society*. Cambridge: Polity.

Brandt, A.M. and Rozin, P. (eds) (1997) *Morality and Health*. London: Routledge.

Bunton, R. (1997) Popular health, advanced liberalism and *Good Housekeeping* magazine, in S. Peterson and R. Bunton (eds) *Foucault, Health and Medicine*. London: Routledge.

Bunton, R., Nettleton, S. and Burrows, R. (eds) (1995) *The Sociology of Health Promotion: Critical Analysis and Consumption*. London: Routledge.

Courtwright, D.T. (1997) Morality, religion and drug use, in A.M. Brandt and P. Rozin (eds) (1997) *Morality and Health*. London: Routledge.

Davis, A.M. (1987) Heart health campaigns, *Health Education Journal*, 39: 74–9.

Davison, C., Frankel, S. and Davey-Smith, G. (1997) The limits of lifestyle: reassessing 'fatalism' in the popular culture of illness presentation, in M. Siddell, (ed.) *Debates and Dilemmas in Promoting Health: A Reader*. Buckingham: Open University Press.

DOH (Department of Health) (1976) *Prevention and Health: Everybody's Business*. London: HMSO.

DOH (Department of Health) (1992) *The Health of the Nation*. London: HMSO.

DOH (Department of Health) (1999) *Saving Lives: Our Healthier Nation*. London: HMSO.

DOH (Department of Health) (2004) *Choosing Health: Making Healthier Choices Easier*. London: HMSO.

Doi, Y. (2005) Health promotion campaign for ethnic minority groups: the case of the radio campaign for Asian populations, in M. King and K. Watson (eds) *Representing Health: Discourses of Health and Illness in the Media*. Basingstoke: Palgrave Macmillan.

Ellis, J. (1999) Television as working through, in J. Gripsrud (ed.) *Television and Common Knowledge*. London: Routledge.

Fairclough, N. (1995) *Media Discourse*. London: Hodder.

Featherstone, M. (1991) *Consumer Culture and Postmodernism*. London: Sage.

Geertz, H.C. (1983) *Local Knowledge*. New York: Basic Books.

Gordon, L. (1997) Teenage pregnancy and out-of-wedlock birth: morals, morality, experts, in A.M. Brandt and P. Rozin (eds) *Morality and Health*. London: Routledge.

Gripsrud, J. (2002) *Understanding Media Culture*. London: Arnold.

Hall, S. (ed.) (1997) *Representation; Cultural Representations and Signifying Practices*. London: Sage.

Hubley, J. (2005) Promoting health in low and middle income countries, in A. Scriven, and S. Garman (eds) (2005) *Promoting Health: Global Perspectives*. Basingstoke: Palgrave Macmillan.

King, M. (2003) Promoting public health: media constructions and social images of health in a post-modern society, in J. Costello, and M. Haggart (eds) *Public Health and Society*. Basingstoke: Palgrave Macmillan.

King, M. and Watson, K. (2001) Transgressing venues: health studies, cultural studies and the media, *Health Care Analysis*, 9(4): 401–13.

King, M. and Watson, K. (eds) (2005) *Representing Health: Discourses of Health and Illness in the Media*. Basingstoke: Palgrave Macmillan.

Koselka, K., Puska, P. and Tuomilheto, J. (1976) The North Karelia Project. A first evaluation, *International Journal of Health Education*, 19: 59–66.

Lalonde, M. (1974) *A New Perspective on the Health of Canadians*. Ottawa: Information Canada.

Leichter, H. (1997) Lifestyle correctness and the new secular morality, in A.M. Brandt and P. Rozin (eds) *Morality and Health*. London: Routledge.

Lefebvre, R.C. (1992) *Social marketing and health promotion*, in R. Bunton and G. MacDonald, (eds) *Health Promotion, Disciplines and Diversity*. London: Routledge.

Lonsdale, J. (2006) Aunty state, *Journal of the Royal Society for the Promotion of Health,* 126(1): 14–15.

Lupton, D. (2003) *Medicine as Culture: Illness, Disease and the Body in Western societies*, 2nd edn. London: Sage.

Lyons, A.C. and Willott, S. (1999) *From Suet Puddings to Superhero: Representations of Men's Health for Women*. London: Sage.

Maibach, E. and Parrott, L. (1995*) Designing Health Messages: Approaches from Communication Theory and Public Health Practice*. London: Sage.

May, T. (1997) *Social Research: Issues, Methods and Process*. Buckingham: Open University Press.

McKee, A. (2003) *Textual Analysis: A Beginner's Guide*. London: Sage.

McKeown, T. (1976) *The Modern Rise of Population*. New York: Academic Press.

Naidoo, J. and Wills, J. (1994) *Health Promotion: Foundations for Practice*. London: Bailliere Tindall.

O'Brien, M. (1995) Health and lifestyle: a critical mess? Notes on the differentiation of health, in R. Bunton, S. Nettleton and R. Burrows (eds) *The Sociology of Health Promotion. Critical Analyses of Consumption, Lifestyle and Risk*. London: Routledge.

Petersen, A.R. (1994) Governing images: media constructions of the 'normal', 'healthy' subject, *Media Information Australia*, 72: 32–40.

Pryce, A. (2005) 'Planting landmines in their sex lives': governmentality, iconography of sexual disease and the 'duties' of the STD clinic, in M. King and K. Watson (eds) *Representing Health: Discourses of Health and Illness in the Media*. Basingstoke: Palgrave Macmillan.

Seale, C. (2003) *Media and Health*. London: Routledge.

Seedhouse, D. (1997) *Health Promotion: Philosophy, Prejudice and Practice*. Chichester: Wiley.

Seedhouse, D. (2003) *Total Health Promotion: Mental Health, Rational Fields and the Quest for Autonomy*. Chichester: Wiley.

Shattuc, J. (1997*) The Talking Cure*. London: Routledge.

Southwell, B. (2000) Audience constructions and AIDS education efforts: exploring communication, assumptions of public health interventions, *Critical Public Health*, 10(3): 314–19.

Stake, R.E. (1998) Case studies, in N. Denzin and Y. Lincoln (eds) *Strategies of Qualitative Inquiry*. London: Sage.

Tones, B.K. (1985) The use and abuse of mass media in health promotion, *Health Education Research, Theory and* Practice, pilot issue: 9–14.

Tones, K., Tilford, S. and Robinson, Y. (1994) *Health Education: Effectiveness and Efficiency*. London: Chapman Hall.

Van Dijk, T.A. (1993) Principles of cultural discourse analysis, *Discourse and Society*, 4: 249–83.

Wallack, L., Dorforman, L., Jennigan, D. and Themba, M. (1993) *Media Advocacy and Public Health, Power for Prevention*. London: Sage.

10 Globalization and public health policy

Jeff Collin and Kelley Lee

The diverse challenges of globalization for public health are being increasingly recognized, and are beginning to transform the institutions and policy actions needed to protect and promote population health. Traditionally public health has been a nationally focused endeavour. While countries have cooperated, particularly since the nineteenth century, to address health issues of international concern, such efforts have been focused within a limited range of institutions and issues, notably the control of selected infectious diseases such as plague, yellow fever and cholera. Collaboration has been primarily through national governments in the form of regulatory controls at national borders, exchange of information, and agreement of common practices and nomenclature. The twentieth century saw a significant expansion of international health cooperation through the activities of the World Health Organization (WHO) and other bodies of the United Nations (UN), bilateral aid agencies and nongovernmental organisations (NGOs). Nonetheless, the main determinants of health continued to be framed as deriving from, and largely confined within, national borders. From this perspective, the mandate of ministries of health and national health systems remained focused on the domestic sphere. By the late twentieth century, this territorially based approach to public health, focused on the state, had been increasingly challenged by processes of globalization (for a background to the history and success of public health in the UK, see Chapter 2 and Chapter 11).

In brief, globalization can be defined as a set of processes leading to more intensive and extensive human interactions across geographical space, notably national borders. Globalization is recognized to have historical roots as far back as the migration of the *Homo* genus from Africa some 1.7 million years ago. The close relationship between the evolution of human societies, and subsequent patterns of health and disease is well documented (Lee 2003). What is distinct within the contemporary world, however, is the reach of globalization processes today, both in its embrace of almost every society and the range of social spheres impacted upon. Contemporary globalization is playing out within the economic, political, cultural and other social spheres, defined by certain values and ideologies, and enabled by the advent of new technologies.

The unprecedented degree and pace of social change resulting from globalization can be understood as having three dimensions. First, there are changes to how individuals and societies define and interact across territorial space. The intensified mobility of populations, the increase in trade relations, and the flow of information and communication across vast distances all challenge the social organization and experience of physical space. Second, there are changes in the perception and experience of time. Many social interactions are being accelerated by the advent of new technologies which enable people to obtain information, carry out day-to-day transactions, and travel across distances faster than previous generations. Third, and perhaps most profoundly, there are changes to the way people perceive themselves and their world. The flow of ideas, beliefs, knowledge and cultural goods across societies is unprecedented, leading to the formation of new social identities which, in some cases, are shared with others and, in other cases, divide individuals and societies from each other. Altogether, spatial, temporal and cognitive changes associated with globalization are impacting on human societies around the world in new and complex ways.

The challenges posed by globalization to public health policy can usefully be understood through the concept of transborder health risk. Put simply, a transborder health risk is a risk to human health that transcends the jurisdictional boundaries of a recognized authority in origin or impact. The authority, acting alone, may have limited capacity to regulate risk, necessitating collaborative efforts across jurisdictional boundaries. The most geographically extensive of these is global health cooperation (for more on the challenges to public health in the context of global cooperation see Lee and Collin 2005; Scriven and Garman 2005).

This chapter examines a number of key areas where globalization poses new challenges for public health policy. Through its impact on varied health determinants and outcomes, globalization requires new ways of thinking about how societies organize to protect and promote population health. For each issue, there is a need to grapple with transborder health risks. At the same time, globalization poses new opportunities for improved collaboration through institution-building, shared knowledge and resources and the creation of a new global public health identity.

Tobacco control

There are several compelling reasons for focusing on tobacco in examining the implications of globalization for UK public health, and here developments in the tobacco pandemic, the tobacco industry and health policy response will be used to highlight the complex intertwining of transborder health risks and opportunities. The necessary starting point from a public health perspective is the sheer scale of tobacco-associated health problems and the inequity of their distribution both globally and nationally. Moreover the trajectory of the tobacco pandemic needs to be understood with reference to the global political economy, as trade liberalization has facilitated expansion by transnational tobacco companies and stimulated rising tobacco consumption in low- and middle-income countries (MICs). Such trends highlight the challenge posed by globalization to health policy, and the WHO's Framework Convention on Tobacco Control (FCTC) provides a particularly striking example of an attempt to develop new forms of health governance in response to globalization (for discussion of tobacco control within the UK, including legislation, see Chapter 17).

Tobacco consumption and health impacts

While global tobacco consumption has increased dramatically over the last two decades, a marked shift in smoking patterns is occurring that has profound implications for health equity. A broad decline in prevalence across most high-income countries over recent decades has coincided with substantial increases among LMICs, with the latter now accounting for an estimated 82 per cent of the world's smokers. This trend is being followed by an inexorable redistribution of tobacco-related disease and death. Around 4.9 million deaths could be attributed to tobacco use in 2000, an increase of 45 per cent over the previous decade, and by 2030 the global toll is expected to reach 10 million, or around one in six adult deaths. The most rapid escalation in tobacco-related mortality has been seen in developing countries, which already account for 50 per cent of such deaths, a proportion expected to rise to 70 per cent by 2030 (Gajalakshmi *et al.* 2000; WHO 2002).

Consumption patterns among LMICs remain strongly differentiated by, among other things, region, product and gender. Though male and female smoking prevalence has broadly converged across much of Europe and North America, there remain huge disparities in tobacco use by gender in many developing countries. World Bank estimates indicate smoking prevalence among men and women in high-income countries at 38 per cent and 21 per cent respectively, contrasting with figures for LMICs of 49 per cent and 9 per cent respectively. China provides a particularly stark example: adult male smoking prevalence of 53.4 per cent contrasting with only 4 per cent among women (Gajalakshmi *et al.* 2000). A combination of broad socioeconomic changes and increasingly targeted marketing by transnational tobacco companies (TTCs) is likely to lead to significant increases in uptake among women, to whom the increased sale of tobacco products has plausibly been described as the single largest product marketing opportunity in the world (Kaufman and Nichter 2001; Asma *et al.* 2005).

Though the tobacco epidemic in the UK is characterized by declining smoking prevalence among men and women, it remains the single greatest cause of preventable illness and premature death. In 2004 smoking was estimated to be responsible for 106,000 deaths each year, down from 120,000 in 1995 (Twigg *et al.* 2004). The health impacts of smoking in the UK are again strikingly inequitable (for further discussion of behaviour, risk and health in relation to inequalities see Chapters 4, 6, 12 and 13). Reductions in smoking rates among lower income groups have lagged far behind those for wealthier ones; around half the difference in survival to 70 years of age between social class I and V is attributable to higher smoking prevalence in class V (Wanless 2004).

Globalization, the tobacco industry and the UK

An important evidence base is emerging documenting the impact of trade liberalization on the tobacco pandemic. The dismantling of obstacles to trade in tobacco by trade agreement, and following regime change in central and eastern Europe, has transformed the tobacco industry, with profound implications for health. The inclusion of agricultural products in the GATT regime after 1994, for example, stimulated substantial expansion in traded tobacco. After a decade of negligible growth, the period from 1994 to 1997 witnessed a 12.5 per cent increase in unprocessed tobacco exports, and cigarette exports grew by 42 per cent between 1993 and 1996 having been relatively stable from 1975 to 1985 (Taylor *et al.* 2000).

The opening of Asian cigarette markets to western-based transnational tobacco companies has been particularly significant in the development of the industry and in stimulating tobacco consumption. The previously closed markets of Japan, Taiwan, South Korea and Thailand, for example, were opened to TTC competition between 1986 and 1990 following pressure from the USA that included the threat of retaliatory trade sanctions. It has been estimated that by 1991 per capita tobacco consumption increased by an average of 10 per cent across these four countries (Chaloupka and Laixuthai 1996). It is important to note the inequitable impacts of trade liberalization on tobacco use. Trade liberalization has led to increased consumption of tobacco overall but, while it has no substantive effect on high-income countries, it has had a big impact on smoking in low-income countries and a significant, if smaller, impact on middle-income countries (Taylor *et al.* 2000).

The UK, with three of the world's five largest tobacco companies, assumes global significance within the contemporary tobacco industry. Imperial and Gallaher have long been dominant within the UK tobacco market, but have addressed the prospect of long-term decline via aggressive expansion strategically focused on LMICs. With the second largest market share behind US-based Philip Morris, British American Tobacco (BAT) is the world's most international tobacco group because of its particular strengths across emerging markets. BAT has undertaken an extensive programme of reorganization and acquisition to exploit the opportunities associated with global change (Collin and Lee 2002), while analysis of corporate documents disclosed following litigation has highlighted the extent to which its global expansion has been strategically dependent on smuggling. Interestingly, a lengthy investigation by the UK Department of Trade and Industry (DTI) into BAT's apparent complicity in contraband came to a quiet demise amid reports of political pressure at the highest levels (Collin *et al.* 2004). This is indicative of at least the partial perpetuation of a historic role of UK governments in promoting the international interests of the tobacco industry (Taylor 1984).

Globalization, health governance and the UK

The nature of the challenge to the nation state's preeminence as the organizational basis for policy has been central to scholarly debates about globalization. Intensified transborder flows are encouraging shifting balances across subnational, national, regional and international levels of governance. Within the UK, devolution has had a profound impact on the character and content of tobacco control policy. The passage of smoke free legislation in England in 2006, for example, provides a remarkable example of policy transfer from the periphery to the centre. Scotland's comprehensive legislation, backed by similar developments in Wales and Northern Ireland and strong pressure from local government, enabled the adoption of measures far in advance of those initially proposed by the Labour government. Legislation prohibiting tobacco advertising and sponsorship similarly illustrates the Europeanization of public policy, though European Union (EU) tobacco control measures have demonstrated the extent to which the pursuit of public health objectives has been subject to the primacy of free trade (Gilmore and McKee 2004; see also Chapter 17).

Arguably the most significant innovation in health governance of the last decade is provided by the Framework Convention on Tobacco Control (FCTC). The first international public health treaty initiated by the WHO, the FCTC constitutes an attempt to develop an appropriate response to globalization and recognition of the inability of traditional health governance to counter effectively the expansion of TTCs. The FCTC negotiations were a core element of then Director General Gro Harlem Brundtland's attempt to revitalize the WHO. They demonstrate considerable success by the WHO in coordinating support from other international organizations, particularly that of the World Bank, for its health-focused agenda. They achieved extensive engagement by member states, requiring considerable interdepartmental consultation and collaboration. Despite substantial conflict over content and development, reflecting tensions between health and other competing objectives, there was an overriding consensus on the value of a framework convention. Finally efforts to situate tobacco control objectives more prominently on related policy agendas including development, human rights and gender represent a partial but significant opening of the policy process to participation by civil society (Collin 2004; for more on the FCTC in the context of tobacco control within the UK, see Chapter 17).

The ambiguity characteristic of the UK Labour government's domestic record on tobacco issues is also evident in its role within the FCTC negotiations. Official support for international tobacco control measures was clearly evident, with both the Departments of Health and International Development making early formal commitments to the FCTC's development. The Secretary of State for Health was given lead responsibility for the negotiations, the Foreign Office having overall responsibility for the conclusion and implementation of its obligations, while the Treasury, the Department of Trade and Industry, sport and regional ministries were recognized as having an interest. Delegations were formally led by the UK's permanent representative in Geneva but were dominated by health officials. The UK was among the most progressive states in recognizing the significance of tobacco control to development, encouraging the European Commission's willingness to use development funds to support tobacco control.

Conversely, however, the UK did not play a prominent supportive role comparable to Canada, New Zealand or Australia, while British contributions caused some unease among advocates for a strong convention. Assessing the UK's contribution is complicated by the opaque and chaotic nature of the EU's role in FCTC proceedings. The European Commission negotiated on behalf of member states in areas covered by European law, while in other areas a common position was typically agreed by member states and advanced by the country holding the presidency. European positions were typically cautious and characterized by a refusal to move beyond the confines of existing EU measures. While attention focused on Germany as the principal brake on EU positions, several member states including the UK were quietly willing to let Germany be the public face of obstructionism (Gilmore and Collin 2002).

To the extent that specifically British concerns could be identified, it appeared that the UK successfully led opposition to the abolition of duty-free sales. The existence of duty-free sales serves both to undermine the effectiveness of taxation in reducing tobacco consumption and to facilitate smuggling, an area in which the British position was perceived by participants as being weak. While the UK never received the opprobrium attached to the USA as a persistent defender of the interests of tobacco companies, it did appear that on such issues the government regarded the interests of UK-based companies as militating against health concerns.

Following four years of negotiations the agreed text of the FCTC received the unanimous endorsement of the 56th World Health Assembly in May 2003. Among the key features of the final text are provisions encouraging countries to enact comprehensive bans on tobacco advertising, promotion and sponsorship; to require large rotating health warnings on packaging that should cover at least 30 per cent of principal display areas, and with provision for pictorial warnings; to prohibit the use of misleading descriptors such as the words light or mild; to increase taxation of tobacco products; to provide greater protection from involuntary exposure to tobacco smoke; and to develop measures to combat smuggling (Hammond and Assunta 2003).

The text is lacking in binding obligations, which may be developed further by a number of issue specific protocols. It also failed to include language that would clarify its status in relation to existing trade agreements, health versus trade being the single most divisive issue during negotiations. Such caveats notwithstanding, however, the final text was both broadly welcomed by health groups and proved to be a remarkable advance on the heavily criticized preceding draft. Along with other EU states, the UK ratified the FCTC in December 2004 (Collin 2004).

Population mobility

Population mobility is a broad term that describes all categories of movement by people, covering where, when and how they move, whether by groups or individuals, whether coerced or voluntary (MacPherson 2001). For descriptive purposes such movements can be crudely classified by duration of travel, UK statistics classifying visits of less than a year as tourism, and migration for those of longer duration, though in fact there is no simple behavioural distinction between tourist and migrant. There is nothing new in noting that international travel has health implications, with the practice of quarantine emerging in Europe as early as the fourteenth century and arguably the most significant global exchange of pathogens occurring via the introduction of diseases to the New World following 1492. The current scale and speed of population mobility suggests, however, that associated transborder health risks are assuming a new salience amid contemporary globalization (for further discussion of population mobility in relation to public health policy, see Chapter 3).

The UK provides an acute example of the rapid intensification of global flows in tourism and migration. UK residents made over 61 million visits abroad during 2003, triple the figure for 1981, while travel to tropical countries is increasing at an annual rate of 8 per cent (HPA 2005a). The UK ranked sixth in the world for international tourism arrivals in 2004 (World Tourism Organization 2005), while the total number of people migrating to the UK reached a record 582,000 in 2004 compared with 360,000 leaving to live elsewhere (ONS 2006).

The impact of population mobility on health is usually understood primarily with reference to infectious disease, and the rapid impact of SARS highlights the continuing, and perhaps increasing, significance of such a focus. This is briefly illustrated below with reference to HIV/AIDS and tuberculosis. But risks associated with population mobility are more extensive, and their diversity in character, duration and range of people affected can be understood using a functional approach to travel health classified across the three phases of pre-departure, journey and destination (Gushulak and MacPherson 2000).

Health risks associated with the pre-departure phase might be particularly acute for refugees, whose flight is often triggered by conflict or disaster situations, but might also encompass the failure of tourists to take adequate precautions against tropical diseases prior to travel. While the most severe risks during the journey itself may be experienced in the context of illegal migration, as in the deaths of 58 Chinese migrants at the port of Dover in 2000, increased attention to occurrences of deep vein thrombosis (DVT) indicate their relevance to tourists. The post-arrival phase demonstrates the long-term and even the cross-generational relevance of population mobility to health status. The persistence of such risks may reflect the lengthy incubation period of a disease such as tuberculosis, experiences of poverty and social exclusion, or hazards associated with subsequent return visits to friends and relatives.

HIV/AIDS

The long association between international travel and the transmission of sexually transmitted diseases (STDs) has assumed a new salience in the context of HIV/AIDS. The arrival of HIV/AIDS in the UK can itself be attributed to travel, and the movements of tourists and migrants continue as factors shaping the epidemiology of the HIV virus.

This is particularly true with respect to heterosexual sex as a means of transmission, now the exposure category for over half of newly diagnosed infections in England and Wales. For those diagnoses where region of probable infection was identified, some 83 per cent of HIV infections attributable to sex between men were acquired within the UK but around 90 per cent of heterosexual infections were acquired elsewhere (HPA 2005a).

Migration from parts of the world with high prevalence of HIV has substantially shaped the epidemic in the UK, with Africa providing the region of probable infection for some 63 per cent of cases acquired by sexual transmission; 77.4 per cent for heterosexual men, 82 per cent for heterosexual women, and less than 3 per cent for homosexual men. The influence of tourism is less clear, though a comparison of country of birth with country of probable acquisition of infection may give a broad indication of its relevance. Some 12 per cent of heterosexual men and women diagnosed were born in the UK, of whom some 45 per cent were probably infected with HIV overseas, notably in sub-Saharan Africa and Thailand (HPA 2005a).

Tuberculosis

Trends in the epidemiology of tuberculosis illustrate how the changing ethnic composition of British society has shaped the distribution of health risks. The long-term nature of risks associated with migration becomes evident from how, within the UK, tuberculosis has become primarily a disease afflicting certain ethnic minorities. In 2003, 70 per cent of tuberculosis cases reported in England, Wales and Northern Ireland were among those born abroad, for whom the tuberculosis rate was 23 times higher than for those born in the UK. The tuberculosis rate for the population as a whole was 12.5 per 100,000, compared with the highest rate of 283 per 100,000 among the black African group, followed by a rate of 124 per 100,000 for the Indian, Pakistani and Bangladeshi group (HPA 2005b; see also Chapter 7).

The relative significance of migration and poverty in explaining the high levels of TB in some of the UK's larger cities remains contested. While migrants are disproportionately evident among high income earners, they are also over-represented among the poor. This experience of poverty can place many migrants and their children in the sort of living and working conditions that are conducive to infection. The high levels of infection among migrants cannot be simplistically attributed to imported infection from the country of origin. A recent study to quantify variation in relative risks of tuberculosis at hospital ward level in Manchester, Liverpool, Birmingham and Cardiff did, however, identify country of birth as the most influential explanatory variable (Bennett *et al.* 2001).

Migration of health professionals

A primary emphasis on health risks associated with heightened population mobility should not detract attention from the opportunities offered by such flows. Such opportunities, however, are often not without controversy, as in the context of treating patients overseas and particularly regarding the migration of health professionals. The health sector provides a clear example of how employers have used migration to address skills shortages, with the National Health Service (NHS) of the UK launching a global advertising campaign to recruit consultants and general practitioners in 2001. The number of newly registered physicians trained overseas doubled by 2003, and from 1997 to 2003 almost three-quarters of the increase in NHS nurses came via international recruitment (Pond and McPake 2006).

While the extent to which the UK benefits from such brain gain is partially offset by the loss of UK-trained professionals, particularly to the USA, the principal impact of such movement is increasingly borne by LMICs. In some countries, such as the Philippines, intended emigration often shapes the decision to train as a nurse and training costs may be offset by remittances (Bach 2003). But in sub-Saharan Africa, in particular, health system capacity has been critically undermined. During 2000, more than 500 nurses left Ghana to work abroad, more than double the number of new nurses graduating in the country that year (Buchan and Sochalski 2004). Increased controversy and policy attention has led to the development of codes of practice, though disputes over the provision of compensation to source countries highlight the constraints imposed by the priority accorded by destination countries to cost-effective recruitment (Bach 2003).

Conclusion

This chapter has examined two broad areas where globalization is creating new challenges and opportunities for public health policy. While focused on the UK, the chapter has relevance for public health policy in other countries. A number of conclusions arise from the above discussion. First, the concept of transborder health risk and opportunity is a useful one for highlighting the positive and negative externalities associated with particular flow variables such as people, goods and services, and information and communication. It is important, however, to frame transborder health risks beyond the threat of infectious diseases from abroad, as focused upon by early forms of international health cooperation. Tobacco control illustrates the ways in which high-income countries can be sources of health risk for LMICs. The issue of population mobility also should not be crudely reduced to fears of infection from foreign nationals. The recent patterns of migration by health professionals, in some cases weakening poorer countries, again demonstrate the complex risks and opportunities created by globalization. Thus risks and opportunities to public health arising from globalization flow in multiple directions and impact on individuals and societies in complex ways. This requires public health policy to adopt a broad conceptualization of the impacts of globalization on health than presently prevails.

Second, this chapter demonstrates that globalization poses a direct challenge to public health systems that have focused efforts at the physical borders of states. Historical fears of infectious diseases, such as cholera and plague, for example, have led to the creation of institutions and practices to protect 'border health'. Ports of entry became natural focal points for such efforts, based on the belief that national borders could be protected by such practices as quarantine and screening. In an age of globalization, such practices may be obsolete and, in some cases, irrational to effective public health practice. There is a need for a paradigm shift, in short, from a fortress approach to protecting the health of populations living within a given geographical location, to one that recognizes the need for policy action both beyond and within jurisdictional boundaries. Given the increasingly porous nature of the territorial borders of all states to an expanding range of health determinants, there is a need to address such factors from a global rather than local perspective.

Third, effectively addressing health challenges posed by globalization requires significant institutional and policy innovation. The issues discussed demonstrate the need for closer cross-sectoral and inter-agency collaboration. Public health policy cannot remain within an institutional silo, but must engage more directly with other sectors and with a broader range of relevant governmental and non-governmental agencies. This requires a wider focus than the traditional notions of health determinants, to include a consideration of how trade, taxation, telecommunications, immigration and transport policies have significant influences on public health outcomes. Moreover, institutional reform is needed beyond the national sphere to embrace new forms of governance at the regional and global levels. The FCTC is a good example of such collaborative effort, ostensibly across governments but also including non-state actors, to advance a clear public health goal. The plethora of institutional arrangements that have emerged in recent years, seeking to protect and promote global health, are an expression of the search for effective governance mechanisms which can address transborder health risks and opportunities.

References

Asma, S., Gupta, P. and Warren, C.W. (2005) Tobacco: the global challenge for health promotion, in A. Scriven, and S. Garman (eds) (2005) *Promoting Health: Global Perspectives*. Basingstoke: Palgrave Macmillan.

Bach, S. (2003) *International Migration of Health Workers: Labour and Social Issues*, working paper. Geneva: International Labour Organization.

Bennett, J., Pitman, R., Jarman, B., Best, N., Alves, B., Cook, A., Hart, D. and Coker, R. (2001) A study of the variation in tuberculosis incidence and possible influential variables in Manchester, Liverpool, Birmingham and Cardiff in 1991–95, *International Journal of Tuberculosis and Lung Disease*, 5(2): 158–63.

Buchan, J. and Sochalski, J. (2004) The migration of nurses: trends and policies, *Bulletin of the WHO*, 82(8): 587–94.

Chaloupka, F. and Laixuthai, A. (1996) *US Trade Policy and Cigarette Smoking in Asia*, working paper No. 5543. Cambridge, MA: National Bureau of Economic Research.

Collin, J. (2004) Tobacco politics, *Development*, 47(2): 91–6.

Collin, J. and Lee, K. (2002) *The United Kingdom, Globalisation and Transborder Health Risk*. London: The Nuffield Trust.

Collin, J., LeGresley E., MacKenzie, R., Lawrence, S. and Lee, K. (2004) Complicity in contraband: British American Tobacco and cigarette smuggling in Asia, *Tobacco Control*, 13(Supp II): ii96–111.

Gajalakshmi, C.K., Jha, P., Ranson, K. and Nguyen, S. (2000) Global patterns of smoking and smoking-attributable mortality, in P. Jha and F. Chaloupka (eds) *Tobacco Control in Developing Countries*. Oxford: Oxford University Press.

Gilmore, A. and Collin, J. (2002) A wake up call for global tobacco control: will leading nations thwart the world's first health treaty? *British Medical Journal*, 325: 846–7.

Gilmore, A. and McKee, M. (2004) Tobacco-control policy in the European Union, in E. Feldman and R. Bayer (eds) *Unfiltered: Conflicts Over Tobacco Policy and Public Health*. Cambridge, MA: Harvard University Press.

Gushulak, B. and MacPherson, D. (2000) Health issues associated with the smuggling and trafficking of migrants, *Journal of Immigrant Health*, 2(2): 67–78.

Hammond, R. and Assunta, M. (2003) The Framework Convention on Tobacco Control: promising start, uncertain future, *Tobacco Control*, 12: 241–2.

HPA (Health Protection Agency) (2005a) *Foreign Travel-associated Illness; England, Wales and Northern Ireland – Annual Report 2005*. London: HPA.

HPA (Health Protection Agency) (2005b) *Annual Report on Tuberculosis Cases Reported in England, Wales and Northern Ireland in 2003*. London: HPA.

Kaufman, N. and Nichter, M. (2001) The marketing of tobacco to women: global perspectives, in J. Samet and S.Y. Yoon (eds) *Women and the Tobacco Epidemic: Challenges for the 21st Century*. Geneva: WHO.

Lee, K. (2003) *Globalization and Health, an Introduction*. London: Palgrave Macmillan.

Lee, K. and Collin, J. (2005) *Global Change and Health*. Maidenhead: Open University Press.

MacPherson, D. (2001) Human health, demography and population mobility, in *Migration and Health*, 1/2001. Geneva: International Organization for Migration.

ONS (Office for National Statistics) (2006) *International Migration: Migrants Entering or Leaving the United Kingdom and England and Wales, 2004*. London: ONS.

Pond, B. and McPake, B. (2006) The health migration crisis: the role of four Organization for Economic Cooperation and Development countries, *The Lancet*, 367: 1448–55.

Scriven, A. and Garman, S. (2005) *Promoting Health: Global Perspectives*. Basingstoke: Palgrave Macmillan.

Taylor, A., Chaloupka, F., Guindon, E. and Corbett, M. (2000) The impact of trade liberalization on tobacco consumption, in P. Jha and F. Chaloupka (eds) *Tobacco Control in Developing Countries*. Oxford: Oxford University Press.

Taylor, P. (1984) *Smoke Ring: The Politics of Tobacco*. London: Bodley Head.

Twigg, L., Moon, G. and Walker, S. (2004) *The Smoking Epidemic in England*. London: Health Development Agency.

Wanless, D. (2004) *Securing Good Health for the Whole Population*. London: TSO.

WHO (World Health Organization) (2002) *The World Health Report 2002: Reducing Risks, Extending Healthy Life*. Geneva: WHO.

World Tourism Organization (2005) *UNWTO Tourism Highlights 2005*. Madrid: UNWTO.

Part 2
Public health action

11 Healthy public policies: rhetoric or reality?

Angela Scriven

This chapter examines both the term and the concept of healthy public policies and their roots and links to the social context of health and to public health promotion strategies, including World Health Organization (WHO) declarations. Developing healthy public policies involves alliances and partnerships that cross sector boundaries of traditional public health policy development and foster a better interaction between personal, social and political arenas. International examples will be used to compare with the UK situation, and explore the extent and effectiveness of healthy public policies to tackle public health targets. A noteworthy exemplar will be the healthy public policy framework used in the Calgary health region in Canada. The Calgary framework will be formulated into a model designed to inform the development of healthy public policies at a local level.

What are healthy public policies?

In the second half of the twentieth century there was a shifting of public health priorities. The shift was brought about initially as a response to both the prevailing resource heavy curative paradigm, as argued in the seminal Canadian public health report authored by Lalonde (1974), the then Minister of Health, and to the demographic trends that were increasing the pressure on the health and welfare services (see Chapter 2 for further discussion of the history of public health policy). In the last two decades of the twentieth century, the public health agenda was also responding to megatrends (Naisbett 1984) that included globalization (see Chapter 10), environmental and social justice issues (Scriven 2005). International organizations such as the WHO responded to these shifting priorities by developing international declarations and charters, through which the need for healthy public policies was identified and disseminated.

The Ottawa Charter (WHO 1986) introduced the principle of healthy public policies and established the building of healthy public policy as a key strategy for population health improvement. In so doing, the Charter intended to make health the responsibility of policy makers in all sectors, and to ensure that the health consequences of policies outside of the health sector had taken account of their health impact. There was a stated need to identify the obstacles to the adoption of healthy public policies in non health sectors and a challenge set to find ways of removing them. At the second International Conference on Health Promotion in Adelaide in 1998, the set of recommendations for healthy public policies went some way to clarifying what the term means and how healthy public policies might be actioned (WHO 1998a).

The Adelaide recommendations refer to healthy public policies as being concerned with health and equity at all levels of policy and accountability for health impact. The aim of healthy public policies is to create supportive environments that make health choices possible or easier so that people can lead healthier lives. Healthy public policies are therefore about making social and physical environments health enhancing. The Adelaide recommendations suggest that in pursuit of healthy public policies, government departments concerned with agriculture, trade, education, industry and communications need to take into account health as an essential factor when formulating policy. Not only this, but that these sectors should be held accountable for the health consequences of their policy decisions. In other words, healthy public policies require health to be incorporated as a fundamental consideration in multi sector policy and have the same importance as economic policy. The Adelaide recommendations assert that four of the health promotion actions in the Ottawa Charter (creating supportive environments for health; strengthening community action for health; developing personal skills; reorientation of health services) are interdependent, but the fifth principle – building healthy public policies – is crucial as it establishes the environment that makes the other four possible (WHO 1998a).

The Adelaide recommendations present a number of arguments that help establish a clearer picture of what a healthy public policy looks like in practice, and from this a number of characteristics of a healthy public policy can be drawn. A healthy public policy:

- assigns high priority to tackling inequalities in health and to underprivileged and vulnerable groups;
- creates supportive environments;
- improves access to health enhancing goods and services;
- recognizes the unique culture of indigenous peoples, ethnic minorities and immigrants;
- promotes equal access to health services;
- responds to the health challenges set by technology, complex ecological interactions and growing international independencies;
- recognizes the link between health and social reform;
- emphasizes consultation and negotiation.

While the characteristics above offer a clearer idea of what a healthy public policy is like, Milo (2001) argues that the meaning of healthy public policies has taken on different hues according to the contexts and the purposes of those who use the term. The following explanations of policy terminology have been developed from the Milo glossary, and attempt to place healthy public policy within other policy constructs.

Policy is a guide to action to change what might otherwise occur, a decision about amounts and allocations of resources that reflect the priorities of decision makers. Policy is therefore a tool to set priorities and guide resource allocation.

Public policy is policy at any level of government. Some levels may have formal or legal precedence over others. Heads of government, legislatures and regulatory agencies empowered by other constituted authorities may set policy. Supranational institutions' policies, as those of the European Parliament, may overrule government policies.

Healthy public policies target the wider determinants of health, through multi-level strategies that might focus on lifestyles/behavioural change, environments, education, information exchange, childcare, transportation, and community and personal social and health services. The fundamental aim is to improve the conditions under which people live.

Policy goals shape the course and pace of change in a preferred direction by influencing actions of public and private organizations, affecting populations, environments and behaviour.

Policy making processes are the political, social and economic processes which shape the content of public policies and healthy public policies. Understanding the nature of these processes can support efforts to strengthen healthy public policies.

Policy stakeholders/players/actors are the people who influence and build policy. These include groups whose status, size (or membership), revenues or activities are affected by current and prospective policies, including political parties, the media, bureaucracies, voluntary and commercial organizations, public interest and professional groups. The notion of communities as the policy stakeholders/players and actors who can and should take action within their immediate environment to improve their own health, or act as an advocate for others, reflects the fundamental ethos of healthy public policies (see www.infonet.st-johns.nf.ca/providers/nhhp/docs/policy.html). Examples of healthy public policies that reflect community participation priorities include international initiatives such as Healthy Cities (see Chapter 16 for a full discussion) and the settings approach to public health (see below and Chapter 15 on workplace settings).

Policy environment refers to the context, including past policy making, socioeconomic conditions, widely expressed values, and population demographics and epidemiology. Periodic scanning of the environment provides clues to what is feasible and timely for healthy public policy initiatives.

Policy instruments are used in policy formulation and include economic, regulatory and educational measures. When the policy climate precludes politically costly instruments, such as raising tax on tobacco, governments can use easier to adopt measures, for example, public health education on the dangers of smoking (see Chapter 17 for a closer examination of the smoking policy environment and smoking policy instruments).

Healthy public policies and the settings approach

Healthy public policies as defined above should therefore create supportive environments and should have components that focus on developing health capacity and social capital at both individual and community levels. As Chapter 6 makes clear, significant public health goals around reducing inequalities in health require the building of social capital. Culture and shared values and belief systems are crucial to social capital, as are education, empowerment and economic and other resources. One of the goals of healthy public policies would be to create high levels of social capital and reduce levels of social inequalities. It has been argued (Bandura 2005) that this is best achieved through a healthy

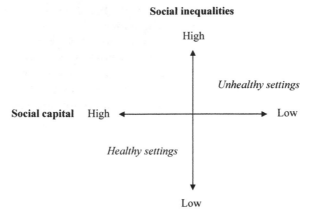

Figure 11.1 Healthy public policies, healthy settings and social capital
Source: adapted from Bandura (2005)

settings approach (see Figure 11.1). Healthy public policies are, therefore, perhaps best understood within the context of healthy settings.

Healthy public policies that are linked to healthy settings embrace the goal of increasing social capital and reflect a move towards:

- strengthening social networks and community cohesion and empowerment;
- participation through partnerships, cooperation and shared decision making within communities and neighbourhoods and with multi-sector agencies;
- a salutogenic ethos where policies are health seeking rather than disease prevention in approach.

Healthy public policies, therefore, are based on democratic concepts involving participation, empowerment and emancipation. These are complex issues and because of this complexity there is likely to be a set of complex policy goals and processes. The links between social capital and income are currently unclear and the debates around the culture of poverty still go on (see Welshman 2006). Nonetheless, it is easy to appreciate why it may be difficult to have trust, confidence and community coherence within an economically unequal community. Because of the complexity of these issues, the development of healthy public policy is as important at the local levels of government as it is nationally and internationally (Nutbeam 2005; Mittelmark 2007).

Public accountability for health is an essential component of healthy public policy. Governments and controllers of resources at a local level are ultimately accountable to their populations for the health consequences of their policies, or lack of policies. A commitment to healthy public policy requires governments to measure and report the health impact of their policies in a language that all groups in society readily understand. As already mentioned, community participation and action is also central to the fostering of healthy public policy and efforts must be made therefore, by policy stakeholders, players and actors, to communicate effectively with those groups most affected by the policy goals.

Evaluating the impact of healthy public policy is also crucial. Health information systems that support this process need to be developed. This will encourage informed decision making for the building of future healthy public policy.

Healthy public policies can also offer a response to the challenges to health set by globalization, involving dynamic and technological changes, complex ecological inter-actions and growing international interdependencies (see Chapter 10 and the discussion of twenty-first-century health challenges later in this chapter). To effectively tackle this, policy efforts require an integrated approach to social and economic development, which firmly establishes the links between health, social and structural reform.

Partners in the healthy public policy process

As outlined above, governments play an important role in population health. Health is also influenced by corporate and business interests, nongovernmental bodies and com-munity organizations. The potential of these other stakeholders to engage in healthy public policy decision making should be encouraged, with trades unions, commerce and industry, academic associations and religious leaders having many opportunities to act in the health interests of the whole community (Mittelmark 2005). In order to embrace healthy public policies, innovatory partnerships must be forged between these stake-holders to provide the impetus for health action (Nutbeam 2005).

If a multi dimensional and holistic definition of health such as the one promoted by the WHO (1946) is accepted, then the boundaries of healthy public policy are broad. The definition of healthy public policy discussed earlier implies that policy decisions are not limited to those relating to healthcare or even other public services. Instead, policy decisions would include a commitment to review all policy actions taken by governments and their public offices and organizations in the light of the impact on health (Mittelmark 2001).

The WHO (1986) identified five basic principles of healthy public policy that expand the connections beyond traditional health and public service responsibilities and in so doing clearly indicate the potential partners in the policy development process:

- economic development must seek to increase quality of life and not just gross national product (GNP);
- the most sensitive indicator of a society's quality of life is the health of its poor and other vulnerable groups (such as children, elders, women who head households, the handicapped, unemployed, migrants and minorities);
- the achievement of equal access to resources for health should be high among the goals of economic development;
- health services cannot alone equalize opportunities for health;
- health equity, health for all, requires the collaboration of all policy sectors, especially those concerned with economics, agriculture and food, education and information, and environment and habitat.

Government constituencies and all the policy stakeholders/players/actors require a broad vision relating to policy goals, which should embrace all of the principles laid out above.

Making public policy healthy

The basic principles of healthy public policy support health promotion and disease prevention as the platforms for individual and population health development. The literature and current practice provide some insight into the range of options for supporting and promoting healthy public policy. For example, healthy public policies often link to the identified primary determinants of disease and illness for a given population, with strategies to reduce disease and promote health and wellbeing specifically targeting the identified causes of ill health.

Other approaches focus on barriers to health within the broader determinants of health for a target population, such as the influence of illiteracy or poverty on obesity. In these cases, a healthy public policy would result in positive changes to inequitable and unhealthy social, economic and/or physical environments.

Another approach is to target the policy at populations of interest, either because of their susceptibility to change, such as children (see Chapter 13), or because of their vulnerable or special situations, such as elderly people.

Whatever policy goals and strategies are adopted, they need to be grounded in both a realistic needs assessment and an ethical health impact assessment (Mittlemark 2007), and to be sustainable.

Finally, policy can relate directly to social capital within communities (Gibson 2007), where disability, gender, ethnicity, age and income differentiation can create social exclusion. If social coherence and inclusion are the foundations for social capital, healthy public policies have an ethical obligation to address these issues.

One way to tackle the challenges of truly embracing healthy public policy is to examine the wellness of policy. Pursuing, at least initially, more local and controllable healthy public policy (Nutbeam 2005) may influence activity within wider population groups and improve the potential for meeting national healthy public policy goals (WHO 1991, 1997, 1998a).

A model for developing healthy public policy

Healthy public policies are one of the strategies used to improve the health of the population in the Calgary region of Canada, using the Adelaide definition of healthy public policy (WHO 1998a) to describe policy that is characterized by an explicit concern for health and equity, and by accountability for health impact. The following is based on the Calgary health region three-dimensional framework, where different components important to building healthy policy are identified and their relationships to one another are implied (see www.calgaryhealthregion.ca/hecomm/pubpolicy/framework.htm). This has been modified for the purposes of this chapter to form a model involving three circles (see Figure 11.2).

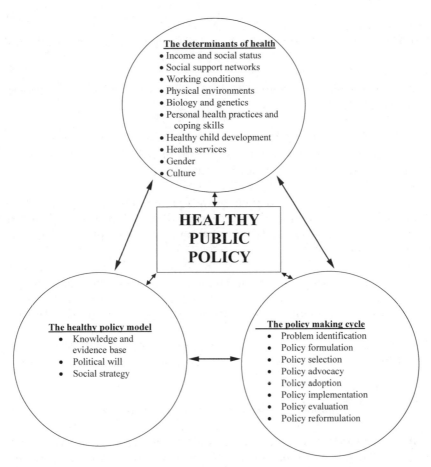

Figure 11.2   Healthy public policy model (adapted from the Calgary framework)

Components of the model

Circle one: the determinants of health

The first component is based on Hamilton and Bhatti's health promotion framework (1996) and contains the determinants of health. This list is critical to the model as it explicitly recognizes that health is created across society and the determinants provide guidance as to the public policy arenas that concern health, including income and education. The determinants of health should inform the breadth of healthy public policy goals, which are:

- to promote the development of public policies that prevent disease;
- to promote the development of public policies that promote health within the context of social, economic and physical environments;
- to promote the development of healthcare policies that reduce inequities in access to health services.

Circle two: the policy making cycle

The second circle is an eight stage policy making cycle that encompasses the following aspects:

1 *Problem identification.* Identification of a need that is a legitimate issue for healthy public policy.

2 *Policy assessment.* Deciding that a policy solution is desirable and a review of all possible policy options, using a spectrum of policy instruments ranging from voluntary to compulsory policy options.

3 *Policy selection.* The process of choosing a preferred policy option. A stakeholder group, following an analysis of the strengths, weaknesses, opportunities and threat of the potential impacts of the various policy options, usually achieves this initial selection.

4 *Policy advocacy.* The process of implementing strategies to inform and persuade. The stakeholder group is often not the group with the authority to adopt policy. The next step frequently is to sell the preferred policy to a decision making body.

5 *Policy adoption.* The processes of adopting the policy. The decision making body may be required to pass motions, have a vote or otherwise to authorize the policy.

6 *Policy implementation.* The process of policy implementation.

7 *Policy evaluation.* The process of monitoring the success of a policy related to specific criteria. This is designed to measure the intended impact of the policy on health and is a critical step in the policy making cycle, necessary to ongoing knowledge development in the policy field.

8 *Policy reformulation.* The process of policy review and revision based on the results of evaluation, environmental changes or new evidence. The policy is revised as needed to improve health outcomes.

Circle three: the healthy policy model

This circle has three areas to be considered in building healthy public policy.

1 *Knowledge and evidence base.* The research related to the significance of the issue and the capacity of a policy solution to improve the problem. Information for the knowledge base may include the literature, demographics, epidemiological data, best practices.

2 *Political will.* Society's desire and commitment to pursue a policy solution. The political will of legislators, administrators, interest groups and the population as a whole will influence the acceptability of various policy options.

3   *Social strategy.* The plan by which the knowledge base and political will is applied in order to build healthy public policy. The social strategy will include how the plan will be sequenced, resourced, communicated and revised. Account will be taken of:
  • links between health impact assessment and healthy public policies;
  • problems with evidence base of effectiveness of healthy public policies;
  • action areas for policy;
  • the need to see health not as an individual problem but as a social one.

The model implies a high degree of interaction between the three circles, reflecting the complexity and the reality of building healthy public policy, with all components seen as important in the process. What is also clear from the model is the close links between healthy public policies and development policies and strategies, such as the Millennium Development Goals with their different domains of environmental planning, education, economic growth, healthcare and employment. Because of these multiple domains, a model such as this necessitates multi agency working and effective collaboration and partnership between all stakeholders (Scriven 2005). This is often complicated by a lack of common language, shared values and set of priorities across the different agencies. There may also be a lack of commitment to community involvement by all of the stakeholders, which is a vital ingredient to successful healthy public policy (Scriven 2007).

The model clearly identifies healthy public policy as targeting the wider determinants of health by putting the issue of health on the agenda of a broad range of public policies. This type of policy requires the development of alliances and partnerships that cross sector boundaries of traditional public policy making, and fosters a better interaction between personal, social and political arenas. In reality, this is complex and fraught with difficulty. While there are some examples of attempts to use healthy public policy as a strategy to promote population health, the rhetoric might be more dominant than any real action or commitment. Chapters 12 and 13 in this text, for example, which provide an overview of the evaluation of Health Actions Zones (HAZs) and of Sure Start in the UK, make clear what the problems are in implementing multi sectoral action. There are some positive points made on HAZs and Sure Start but generally there is no consensus view on how successful such complex multi agency programmes and healthy public policy initiatives can be.

Healthy public policies and twenty-first-century health challenges

The Ottawa Charter gave birth to the idea of healthy public policy and was also the first health strategy to express the notion of modernity, by presenting the view that health is created in the context of everyday life, where people live, love, work and play (WHO 1986); hence, as discussed earlier, the perception that settings are the area where healthy public policies are most effective and visible. There has, however been a significant development since Ottawa in the way societies are shaping themselves into active communities and active individuals that form part of the social environment to which healthy public policies relate.

In many ways the health challenges in the twenty first century are similar to those that came before, with an abundance of environmental health risks and non-communicable and communicable disease to confront (Davey 2005; Kickbusch and Seck 2007). What has changed is the social context in which public health action takes place, as the chapters in Part 1 of this book effectively demonstrate. There are also health issues to contend with that relate specifically to the social context, such as increased longevity (see Chapter 3) and global security risks (Middleton and Sidel 2007).

Significant technological advancements have also changed the way people communicate and spend their time and money. Healthy public policies need therefore to take account of the new challenges brought on by the changing social context of health. Empowerment in the consumer society, for example, requires consumer and citizen competencies, in a media-dominated (see Chapter 9), globalized world (see Chapter 10) where transboundary action is fundamentally important. The notion of supportive environments also becomes more complex in an evolving society, with rapid flows of people (Nutbeam 2005; Kickbusch 2006). Active citizenship has never been more crucial to healthy public policies and empowerment is a prerequisite of active citizenship. In the twenty first century, global citizenship will be paramount. What are crucial to take healthy public policies forward are the empowerment principles and the enabling, mediating, advocating competencies that were embedded in the Ottawa Charter.

There has also been a shifting of power with new health activists emerging that are motivating and shaping healthy public policy in a dynamic manner. The cult of celebrity has introduced a plethora of health policy stakeholders, players and actors, such as Jamie Oliver in the UK, shaping food, nutrition and health policy as they relate to schools, Bill Gates as a global philanthropist tackling the major global health inequality issues and pop musicians appearing to be able to exert more influence than politicians over transnational health policy relating to aid and AIDS.

Given the changes to the social contexts and the introduction of new types of health policy activist outlined above, Nutbeam (2005) has argued that the concepts of healthy public policy as laid out in Ottawa need to evolve. This evolution, he argues, is necessary in order that more effective policy action can be taken to mitigate the negative impact on health of globalization and also to harness the positive benefits that flow from economic development and improvements in access to material resources. This should include innovatory partnerships with private-sector organizations, as suggested earlier in this chapter. Nutbeam also suggests that the basic concept of healthy public policy should be reinterpreted to make it more relevant for the diverse range of political and governance structures present globally.

The evolution suggested by Nutbeam might see a reinvigoration of health policy processes and an emergence of healthy public policy as a central approach in the repertoire of strategies for public health.

There are a number of conclusions that can be drawn from this assessment of healthy public policies as a strategy for addressing the social context of health. The most important deduction is that healthy public policy can be seen both as a process and as an ethos and a principle that reflects joined up thinking. It is clear that the rhetoric of healthy public policy is strong and is influencing decision making at international, national and local levels. Joined up thinking is now strongly embraced by political leaders, and it is generally regarded as fundamentally important that health impact assessment permeates across the policy arenas. The process of developing and implementing healthy public policy appears to be less defined however, and this can only lead to the conclusion that the rhetoric is stronger than the reality.

Healthy public policy endeavour has also arguably been sporadic and limited compared to the overall rhetoric. Much of the public health related policy in the UK, for example, has often reverted to practice around health education targeting behavioural and lifestyle choices related to healthy living, rather than tackling the broader determinants through multi sectoral action. Clearly there have been shifts over the past decade, with neighborhood renewal and other community development initiatives (see for example Chapter 14) demonstrating the will to broaden the public health policy agenda. The examples contained within the public health action part of this book, such as HAZs (Chapter 12), Sure Start (Chapter 13) and the settings approach exemplified by the Healthy Workplaces (Chapter 15) and Healthy Cities (Chapter 16) initiatives go some way to indicate the potential for healthy public policies, but also demonstrate the difficulties involved with such complex policy innovations. It is hoped that the examples being set in regions such as Calgary will pave the way for more rigorous updating and application of the healthy public policy principles contained in the Ottawa Charter.

References

Bandura, B. (2005) Social capital and health. Paper presented at the conference Health Promotion in Higher Education in the Light of the Bologna Process, 22–23 September, Szeged, Hungary.

Davey, B. (2005) Key global health concerns for the twenty-first century, in A. Scriven and S. Garman (eds) *Promoting Health: Global Perspectives*. Basingstoke: Palgrave Macmillan.

Gibson, A. (2007) Does social capital have a role to play in the health of communities? In J. Douglas, S. Earle, S. Handley, C.E. Lloyd and S. Spurr (eds) *A Reader in Promoting Public Health: Challenge and Controversy*. London: Sage.

Hamilton, N. and Bhatti, T. (1996) *Population Health Promotion: An Integrated Model of Population Health and Health Promotion*. Ottawa: Health Promotion Development Division.

Kickbusch, I. (2006) Ottawa – challenges we face. Talk given to the UK Health Promotion Academics Network on 28 November at the OU London Office.

Kickbusch, I. and Seck, B. (2007) Global public health, in J. Douglas, S. Earle, S. Handley, C.E. Lloyd and S. Spurr (eds), *A Reader in Promoting Public Health: Challenge and Controversy*. London: Sage.

Lalonde, M. (1974) *A New Perspective on the Health of Canadians*. Ottawa: Information Canada.

Milo, N. (2001) Glossary: healthy public policy, *Epidemiology and Community Health*, 55: 622–3 (September).

Middleton, J. and Sidel, V.W. (2007) Terrorism and public health, in J. Douglas, S. Earle, S. Handley, C.E. Lloyd and S. Spurr (eds) *A Reader in Promoting Public Health: Challenge and Controversy*. London: Sage.

Mittelmark, M. (2001) Promoting social responsibility for health: health impact assessment and healthy public policy at the community level, *Health Promotion Intenational*, 16(3): 269–74.

Mittelmark, M. (2005) Global health promotion: challenges and opportunities, in A. Scriven, and S. Garman (eds) *Promoting Health: Global Perspectives*. Basingstoke: Palgrave Macmillan.

Mittelmark, M. (2007) Promoting social responsibility for heath: health impact assessment and healthy public policy at the community level, in J. Douglas, S. Earle, S. Handley, C.E. Lloyd and S. Spurr (eds) *A Reader in Promoting Public Health: Challenge and Controversy*. London: Sage.

Naisbett, J. (1984) *Megatrends: Ten Directions Transforming Our Lives*. London: Future Macdonald.

Nutbeam, D. (2005) What would the Ottawa Charter look like if it were written today? *RHP&EO, The Electronic Journal of the International Union for Health Promotion and Education*, www.rhpeo.org/reviews/2005/19/index.htm (accessed 19 December 2006).

Scriven, A. (2005) Promoting health: a global context and rationale, in A. Scriven and S. Garman (eds) *Promoting Health: Global Perspectives*. Basingstoke: Palgrave Macmillan.

Scriven, A. (2007) Developing local alliance partnerships through community collaboration and participation, in S. Handsley, C.E. Lloyd, J. Douglas and S. Spurr (eds) *Policy and Practice in Promoting Public Health* London: Sage.

Welshman, J. (2006) Searching for social capital: historical perspectives on health, poverty and culture, *The Journal of the Royal Society of Health*, 26(6).

WHO (World Health Organization) (1946) *Constitution of the World Health Organization*. Geneva: WHO.

WHO (World Health Organization) (1986) Ottawa Charter for Health Promotion. Geneva: WHO.

WHO (World Health Organization) (1991) *Sundvall Statement on Supportive Environments for Health*. Geneva: WHO.

WHO (World Health Organization) (1997) *The Jakarta Declaration on Health Promotion in the 21st Century*. Geneva: WHO.

WHO (World Health Organization) (1998a) *The Adelaide Recommendations (WHO/HPR/HEP/ 95.2)*. Geneva: WHO.

WHO (World Health Organization) (1998b) *Health for All in the 21st Century* (A51/5). Geneva: WHO.

12 Health Action Zones: multi-agency partnerships to improve health

Linda Bauld and Mhairi Mackenzie

Health Action Zones (HAZs) were the first area-based initiative introduced by the New Labour government following its election victory in 1997. They were multi-agency partnerships located in some of the most deprived areas of England that aimed to improve health and reduce health inequalities by investing in projects and programmes to address the determinants of health as well as improve local health services. The initiative existed between 1998 and 2003 and was the subject of a national evaluation funded by the Department of Health (DoH) (Barnes *et al.* 2005; Bauld *et al.* 2005a). This chapter outlines key elements of the development of HAZs and provides an insight into the change processes undertaken and the impact of the initiative.

Background

In May 1997, the then Secretary of State for Health, Frank Dobson, announced his intention to establish a number of HAZs in England. These would be pilot projects aiming 'to explore mechanisms for breaking through current organizational boundaries to tackle inequalities, and deliver better services and better health care, building upon and encouraging cooperation across the NHS' (DoH 1997: 145). The guidance made it clear that successful zones would create alliances for change by harnessing the dynamism of local people and organisations and building on the success of area based regeneration partnerships. Partnership working would provide added impetus to the task of tackling ill health and reducing inequalities in health. The guidance also stated that HAZ status would provide opportunities for the modernization and reshaping of health and social services. HAZs were asked to adopt seven underlying principles in their plans and activities:

- achieving equity;
- engaging communities;
- working in partnership;
- engaging front-line staff;
- taking an evidence based approach;
- developing a person-centred approach to service delivery;
- taking a whole systems approach.

In October 1997 the DoH invited health authorities in conjunction with local authorities and other agencies to submit bids to become HAZs. The DoH received 41 bids from 49 health authorities. From these HAZ status was granted to 11 areas from April 1998 (DoH 1998a). Of those areas not selected in the first wave, a number were asked to submit further applications, and 15 more areas were granted HAZ status from April 1999 (DoH 1999).

The 26 HAZs were located in diverse areas of England. They were mainly concentrated in the North and Midlands, with four zones in London, one in the Home Counties and two in the south west. In total, the HAZs included 34 health authorities and 74 local authorities. However, the organizational configuration varied significantly between zones (Judge *et al.* 1999). Some HAZs were relatively small (such as Luton, with a population of 200,000) while others were large conurbations (such as Merseyside with a population of 1.4 million). Overall, HAZ areas covered a third of the English population. The total amount of resources made available to HAZs is difficult to estimate precisely because money was available in a variety of different forms for various purposes. Resources for specific activities such as innovation projects or for drug prevention and smoking cessation supplemented programme funding. It is estimated that, on average, HAZs received funding of approximately £4–5 million per year at 2004 prices. This represented a very modest injection of additional resource in relation to the size of health and local authority budgets, but it was intended to provide a change management fund that would promote reform in existing services.

HAZ activities

In order to address the health needs of their varied populations, HAZs chose to invest in a wide range of projects and programmes. These aimed to address the range of factors that can shape and influence health, from poor housing and unemployment to inequitable access to healthcare and inadequate service provision. Initial information regarding these activities was provided in the HAZ implementation plans that were produced by each partnership at the start of the initiative. These plans were then modified following feedback from the DoH and adapted locally as each zone developed.

A total of 214 programmes were identified in the initial HAZ plans (Judge *et al.* 1999). Each programme was allocated to one of seven major categories according to its main focus. These were:

- population groups;
- health problems;
- determinants of health;
- health and social care;
- community empowerment;
- internal processes;
- mixed.

Almost a sixth of the work programmes (34 in total) related primarily to improving the health of particular population groups. Of these, around half focused on young people, but a number of others targeted older people, black and minority ethnic groups and parents. A further 28 programmes related to a specific health problem. The biggest group of programmes in this category focused on mental health as a priority. The remainder covered a range of issues such as accidents and violence, cardiovascular disease, diabetes, physical disabilities and others.

In line with the HAZ focus on a social model of health, the largest proportion of initial programmes, almost a third, a total of 61, were aimed at addressing the determinants of health, including improving employment, housing, education, tackling substance abuse, and promoting opportunities to engage in healthy lifestyles. The programmes that concentrated on health and social care accounted for just over a tenth of initial HAZ activity. Many of these related particularly to improving primary care or community services, and a smaller number to hospital services and health promotion. A further tenth of programmes were centred on involving local communities, and another group focused on the process of HAZ development, including strategy, partnership-building and local evaluation. Finally, there were a small number of 'mixed' programmes that combined a range of approaches.

Within these initial programmes, more than 2000 separate projects or activities were identified. As the initiative developed, the focus of programmes and projects changed in some HAZs due to local or national factors (Bauld *et al.* 2001). But the complexity and range of HAZ ambitions did not. In fact, the evaluation concluded there was hardly any aspect of population health improvement or community regeneration that at least one of the HAZs was not concerned with in one way or another (Judge and Bauld 2006).

The national evaluation

A detailed description of the approach taken to the national evaluation of HAZs is provided elsewhere (Judge *et al.* 1999; Mackenzie and Benzeval 2005; Judge and Bauld 2006). Here we summarize the initial tender requirements of the DoH for the evaluation and describe the shape of the framework that was developed to learn from such a complex intervention.

In 1998 the DoH released a bid for the evaluation that was extremely broad in scope (DoH 1998b). The successful evaluators were, for example, to cover a range of strategic themes of contemporary policy relevance, to assess both processes and impact and, crucially, to take a development role in the establishment of HAZs as learning organizations. In this respect the HAZ evaluation represented the new breed of approach to policy learning that was encouraged by New Labour (Martin and Sanderson 1999).

In our bid for the evaluation we outlined four principles that were instrumental in shaping our approach. These were as follows. First, a theories of change approach, as devised by the Aspen Institute (Connell *et al.* 1995; Fulbright-Anderson *et al.* 1998) was thought to represent the best opportunity to learn about what particular HAZ strategies were most successful in which sets of contexts. In particular, since we would be unable to capture changes at the level of long term health goals within a short term evaluation, this approach would help to determine if intermediate outcomes were consistent with achieving sustainable change in the future. Second, the potential for policy contamination was expected to render a controlled design unfeasible. Third, it was anticipated that the collection of monitoring data (involving several rounds of fieldwork with HAZ project managers) across all HAZs would augment a more focused case study design. Fourth, it was argued that the national approach should be informed by a partnership ethos. This indicated a commitment to sharing evaluation tools, supporting a learning network and providing formative feedback regularly to local areas.

The complexity of the HAZ programme led us to believe that a modular approach to the evaluation would be the most effective means of learning about the kinds of changes brought about by its implementation in a variety of local settings. An almost infinite number of ways of categorizing the intervention could have been invented but the approach we adopted derived from our understanding of what it was that HAZs were trying to achieve. The broad change pathway that we believed lay at the heart of the programme was that, through developing collaborative capacity within partnerships and communities local areas would create the momentum for sustainable whole systems change that would in turn lead, in the longer term, to improved population wellbeing and reduced health inequalities. Three case study modules were devised to focus on these elements of the pathway. The fourth module of the evaluation monitored change and provided developmental support across all HAZs.

As well as a focus on the a priori issues, tackled through the modular approach, the evaluation as it progressed also invested effort in assessing how the sum of HAZ activities and processes made a difference within their short lifespan. This was achieved in two main ways. First, we tried to determine whether the initiative had made any impact on population health. Second, we drew on the perceptions of key stakeholders regarding the impact of HAZs.

The remainder of the chapter focuses on two questions: what were the factors influencing whether HAZs were able to contribute to whole systems change in relation to influencing the social determinants of health; and, using the broadest interpretation of impact, what did HAZs contribute? More detailed findings in relation to both of these questions as well as those relating to the kinds of collaborative capacity built by HAZs and their approaches to tackling health inequalities can be found in Barnes *et al.* (2005).

Factors influencing whole systems change

To make sustainable inroads into tackling the social determinants of ill health at a local level HAZs needed to embed a broad public health agenda within health and local authority planning structures. This section describes what is meant by a whole systems model of change and explores the factors perceived to influence how far eight case study HAZs progressed in bringing about such change.

Whole systems thinking derives largely from management literature (Bertalanffy 1952; Checkland 1981; Checkland and Scholes 1990) and is suited to the evaluation of the kinds of initiatives developed under New Labour since these explicitly rest on the development of multi agency partnerships to tackle complex social problems (Barnes *et al.* 2005). The model of whole systems change used in the HAZ evaluation derived from that of Stewart *et al.* (1999). This contends that all stages in the change process, from initial consultation and capacity building through to evaluation, are highly interrelated, and that successful area-based programme development, implementation and sustainability rely on coherent approaches at both national and local levels. In relation to HAZs, the focus was the national and local factors impacting on three key elements of the change process: strategy development, approaches to learning about the impacts of investments, and purposeful efforts to mainstream change (Mackenzie *et al.* 2005).

Strategy development

Case study HAZs believed that there were three main factors at a national level that impacted on their ability to develop and implement effective strategies aimed at tackling the social determinants of health. These were: the extent to which the national policy context was conducive to the approaches that HAZs wished to adopt; whether there was a stability of intent in relation to the HAZ initiative; and, related to this, whether political leadership remained focused on the goal of tackling health inequalities. In reality the policy context in the early days was thought to be broadly in line with HAZ assumptions. For example, programmes for children and young people launched across policy domains were in keeping with the view that socioeconomic deprivation in the early years leads to long term health and social disadvantage. On the other hand, a change in ministerial leadership for health and a growing government focus on service modernization brought with them a very real sense that the focus for HAZs was shifting from the development of innovative and bottom up solutions to local health inequalities to the achievement of national targets.

At a local level some of the factors that served to best buffer HAZ strategies from these changing directives were: strong local leadership; purposeful efforts to develop local collaborative capacity; and strategic approaches to investment. A small number of the case study HAZs, for example, were driven by charismatic individuals who viewed collaboration with partner organizations and local communities as not only a necessary condition of changing services but as a process requiring investment in its own right. Furthermore, there was a widely held view that change had been driven most effectively where a strategic commissioning approach was taken to the development of new pieces of work as opposed to the funding of a myriad of projects through a bidding process.

Approaches to evaluation and learning

Within a whole systems model reflection, learning and evaluation are the ways in which the system regulates itself and adjusts to its changing context (Stewart *et al.* 1999). Within case study HAZs a number of factors affected whether learning was generated that could contribute to these processes.

At a national level, three main strengths of the HAZ context could be identified. First, there appeared to be a genuine commitment to both national and local evaluation and to collaboration between the two. The initiatives were set up as learning organizations and the national evaluation was encouraged to share tools and approaches with evaluation colleagues at a local level. This commitment was demonstrated through the funding of HAZNet, a web based system to promote the transfer of learning across and within individual HAZs. Support for evaluation was also demonstrated through the funding of a national fellowship scheme whereby practitioners could receive small-scale resources to conduct research and/or development activities relating to their own area of work.

In addition to these three factors the rhetoric of New Labour's evidence-based policy agenda was also supportive of learning through its focus on what works (Davies *et al.* 2000). However, what works was viewed locally as a double edged sword, as a means of disengaging from ineffective practice as well as a means of stifling HAZs' innovation agenda. A further contentious tool in the national armoury to encourage evaluation and learning was its performance monitoring system. This required local HAZs to provide high-level statements stating their goals, activities, anticipated outputs, performance indicators and outcomes. This information was used to grade individual initiatives. Few HAZs found this a useful way of representing their strategic intent or progress and many were sceptical about how and if the data were used at a policy level other than to provide summary judgements.

Despite their very skewed presentation of what HAZs were doing and why, the high-level statements did provide a partial means of gaining an overview of the planning and monitoring process within individual areas. They suggested that in general HAZs had difficulty in producing logical plans that linked their main goals to doable strategies that could be measured using pre specified outcomes and indicators. In other words, the doability and testability of their strategies were often seriously flawed (Judge and Bauld 2001; Judge and Mackenzie 2002). This finding chimes with those emerging from the evaluation of other complex initiatives (Herbert and Anderson 1998; Mackenzie and Blamey 2005) and suggests that, while good planning is important and support for planners required (Killoran and Popay 2002), there is something about the inherent complexity of multi agency solutions to problems that is inimical to detailed specification of programmes at the micro level (Barnes *et al.* 2003).

At the local level there were a number of additional factors that impacted on HAZs' capacity to learn. First, there was considerable variation in the commitment given to learning as a process. In some areas evaluation was a significant strategic investment from the beginning with evaluability built into programme development, in others it was an add on late in the day. The case study HAZs also took different approaches to evaluation. In some the primary focus was on collecting monitoring data, in others building capacity for learning at a project level predominated. A small number developed strategic evaluation frameworks at the beginning of the initiative that allowed them to integrate learning generated at different levels within the overall HAZ system. These were in the best position to provide a connected assessment of progress (Wilkinson and Appelbee 1999; Chapman 2002).

Mainstreaming

As with other area-based initiatives HAZs were time limited. Consequently, to sustain their investments and developments, resources and commitments at a local level needed to be secured. What were the national-level factors that were perceived to impact on their ability to mainstream locally? First, the likelihood of gaining support from local partners was thought to have been compromised by the national message that HAZ funding would not be continued as initially planned and by the development of new policies that were absorbing government energies. Second, organizational developments within two key elements of the whole system for tackling social determinants of health (primary care and the local authorities) also threatened to marginalize HAZs, and the degree to which joined up government had been practised was questioned. It was not clear to some HAZs, for example, whether plans for the new Primary Care Trusts and Local Strategic Partnerships would compromise broad public health approaches to tackling health inequalities (Benzeval 2005). Finally, the extent to which national policy makers had created the space to mainstream policy learning from the HAZ initiative was called into question by the fact that decisions about future funding were being taken prior to the completion of the national evaluation. This challenge to an evidence-based policy making culture is well documented (Weiss 1998; Young *et al.* 2002; Nutley *et al.* 2003; Sanderson 2004; Mackenzie *et al.* 2006).

At a local level HAZs varied in the extent to which they were able to develop mainstreaming strategies. First they differed in whether mainstreaming was planned for at the beginning of the initiative or whether it was a reactive response to the realization that funding would not continue indefinitely and may end sooner than anticipated. Pluye and colleagues (2004, 2005) argue convincingly that, to be successful, sustainability is a process that should be explicit at the strategy development stage. Those case study HAZs that built strategic decision making processes into their planning cycle confirm the analysis that this was the most likely way of sustaining the HAZ way of working. Furthermore, those that took a broad view of mainstreaming, to include the sustaining of practice and policies as well as individual projects (Stewart *et al.* 2002) reported greater successes. HAZs also varied in the extent to which they saw fledgling governance arrangements at a local level to be a threat to their endeavours; those who did not tended to take a dynamic view of partnership that assumed that organizations would always be in a degree of flux and that renegotiating approaches is an integral part of systems change.

In summary, a whole systems change model was a helpful way of conceptualizing differences between HAZs in terms of their ability to progress the broad public health agenda and to plan for health improvement. The key factors at both national and local level that affected progress are summarized in Table 12.1. The HAZs most effective in impacting on the whole system were those that maintained a clear focus on their strategic approach, set up frameworks for learning from their activities and built mainstreaming processes into their ways of working.

Table 12.1 Factors impacting on the change process

Stage of change process	National-level factors	Local factors
Strategy development	• Conducive policy context • Clarity of purpose and sustained focus on aims of programme at national level • Political leadership	• Clarity of purpose • Leadership • Capacity for collaboration • Approaches to strategy implementation
Evaluation and learning	• Commitment to national and local evaluation • Capacity-building • Fostering networks	• Planning and monitoring • Commitment to local evaluation • Capacity-building

	• 'What works' and innovation • Monitoring systems	• Learning across the organization
Sustainability	• Maintained commitment to programme • Joined-up governance • Structures for policy learning	• Focus on the mainstream • Dynamic partnerships

Impact

The modular approach to the national evaluation meant that conclusions about impact were drawn in relation to the key themes of the study described above, including whole systems change. The evaluation did, however, also attempt to assess the extent to which the sum of HAZ activities and processes made a difference within their short lifespan. This was achieved in two main ways. First, we tried to determine whether the initiative had made any impact on population health. Second, we drew on the perceptions of key stakeholders regarding the impact of HAZs.

Population health

HAZs were expected to make a significant contribution to improving population health in their area. However, relatively little thought was given to how outcomes would be measured. The DoH did not require HAZs to collect a common dataset. In addition, the national evaluation was not commissioned (or resourced) to use traditional evaluation tools (such as household surveys across HAZs) to measure any changes between baseline and follow up through time. Thus attempting to measure changes in population health through primary data collected for local or national evaluation was not possible.

Given that there were no HAZ-specific data for measuring the impact of the initiative, the evaluation team identified appropriate routinely collected statistics that could shed some light on changes in population health through time. One of the best sources of this type of data is the *Compendium of Clinical and Health Indicators,* which is commissioned by the DoH and produced by the National Centre for Health Outcomes Development (NCHOD). We selected a range of indicators from the *Compendium* with the objective of identifying whether there was a demonstrable difference between HAZ and non-HAZ areas. At the time of conducting the analysis, the latest available data related to the year 2001/2. We took as the baseline 1997/8 data, the year before the first wave of HAZs was established.

Data were analysed for a range of health indicators relevant to HAZ activities. This included all cause mortality for different age groups, mortality from coronary heart disease, mortality from suicide and mortality from accidents and accidental falls. There are limitations associated with each of these indicators that we describe elsewhere (Bauld *et al.* 2005b). The analysis was conducted in order to obtain the percentage change in each indicator between 1997/8 and 2001/02. This was calculated for four groups, local authorities in first-wave HAZs and second-wave HAZs, the most deprived non HAZ local authorities, and non deprived non HAZ local authorities. The percentage change for the whole of England was also calculated for each indicator (Bauld *et al.* 2005b).

Findings from the analysis were mixed. Overall, HAZs appeared to have out-performed other areas in relation to a number of indicators that are related to their programmes and national policy priorities. First-wave HAZs in particular, which had an extra year to make an impact, appeared to have seen more positive changes in relation to all cause mortality and coronary heart disease mortality than other areas. Findings were however not consistent between indicators. Mortality from suicide increased in all areas, with the largest increase in first-wave HAZs. This is despite the existence of some HAZ programmes focusing on addressing the causes of suicide, particularly among young men. In addition, second-wave HAZs and deprived non HAZ local authorities saw a decrease in mortality and accidents from falls, while all other areas increased. This is despite the fact that several first-wave HAZs had projects with an accident prevention focus.

What this analysis suggests is that, at best, and within a short time frame, HAZs may have made some positive contribution to health improvement. But it was limited and may well have had little or nothing to do with HAZ activities but instead be due to other factors or initiatives that were implemented at the same time. This type of analysis of routinely available statistics fails to shed much light on the many different ways in which the HAZ endeavour made a difference to local people and agencies. To gather this equally valid perception of impact the evaluation team sought the views of those working in HAZs.

Perceptions of impact

A range of key stakeholders in 8 of the 26 HAZs were interviewed in 2003 and asked to provide examples of elements of HAZ work that they defined as successful, in addition to exploring barriers and limits to success (Sullivan *et al.* 2004). They provided examples of individual projects or activities and explained the type of evidence they used to define successful interventions. They also described what individual projects and processes had achieved. These achievements were closely related to the overall principles or objectives of HAZs. The list of achievements is outlined in Table 12.2.

Table 12.2 Achievements of HAZs

1 Introducing a non medical perspective to health
2 Getting important health related issues onto local agendas
3 Encouraging closer working relationships between health and social services
4 Creating infrastructure for sustainable partnership working
5 Precipitating a culture/attitude shift via the 'HAZ way of working'
6 Facilitating change to/introduction of mainstream services
7 Stimulating the involvement of the public as citizens and users
8 Facilitating shared learning
9 Enabling experimentation

Some successful HAZ activities were credited with introducing a non medical perspective to health. HAZs were described as stimulating debate amongst stakeholders about what it means to be healthy and as challenging the dominant medical model of health through the introduction of social perspectives, as well as raising awareness of the wider determinants of health.

Likewise HAZ activities were described as contributing to raising the profile of important health-related issues and getting them onto the agenda of a range of local agencies. Here HAZs were often cited as playing the role of champion, profiling issues or the needs of groups that in other circumstances may have been marginalized. In addition to projects enabling vulnerable groups to receive improved support, HAZs also facilitated links with partners outside health and in some cases helped to secure the profile of these issues/groups in developing community strategies.

HAZ activities were also credited with achieving a range of local changes that related to improved relationships between agencies and improved ways of working. This included encouraging closer working relationships between health and social services. This was particularly significant when it involved aspects of both services that had traditionally not worked together, for example, engaging education colleagues in health-promoting activities. In addition HAZs were credited with preparing the ground for lasting partnership working in each area. Professionals argued that HAZs provided the necessary infrastructure and framework for coordinating the activities of a range of organizations. HAZ impact here was important both in terms of creating effective mechanisms for delivering changes in relation to health and in some cases in providing a template for the development of Local Strategic Partnerships.

Furthermore, local stakeholders cited HAZs as influencing the way in which key players related to each other. This was described as leading to a culture or attitude shift. Several professionals referred to long-standing tensions between health authorities and local authorities in their area and the contribution made by HAZs to overcoming these.

These changed relationships in turn were described as contributing to the emergence of an HAZ way of working, an acknowledgement that changing health outcomes was a collective endeavour and that innovation could emerge from cross sectoral interaction. Testament to the local change wrought by HAZs was the fact that a wide range of partners continued to attend HAZ coordinating meetings even though there might not be any immediate benefit for them.

Another achievement that was described was a change to mainstream services in several of the eight HAZs. Professionals argued that HAZ projects or processes had influenced service delivery. In some cases these changes were described as a HAZ contribution to the modernization of mainstream services. This was particularly relevant as modernization was intended to be one of the underpinning principles of the initiative as a whole.

Successful HAZ projects and activities were also described as stimulating the involvement of the general public as citizens and service users. HAZs gave key service providers the means to test out how to involve service users and local communities. Some HAZ activities were also credited with facilitating shared learning locally. Learning was highlighted in relation to two themes in particular: learning about the difficulties associated with working in partnership and identifying ways to overcome these, and learning about what works in terms of service change and innovation.

Finally, stakeholders argued that, within their short lifespan, HAZs had to some extent enabled experimentation. The development of particular projects and activities was considered to have granted local partners the freedom to act. HAZ funding provided an opportunity to try new things without having to demonstrate how they contributed to overall organizational objectives or national targets. This was particularly the case in the first few years of HAZ funding. The resources provided were described as a safety net, meaning that local actors believed that existing services and practices would not necessarily be jeopardized if the HAZ experiment failed.

In concluding, it is important to reiterate that within their relatively short lifespan, HAZs developed ambitious plans to improve health and reduce health inequalities in England by addressing the wider determinants of health. Evidence regarding their contribution to health improvement is mixed, but this is as much a product of their abbreviated life and the political and structural changes they encountered as their inability to realize their initial objectives. HAZs varied in the extent to which they were able to achieve whole systems change but some made considerable progress towards developing local partnerships and processes to support the change process and ensure some sustainability. This is supported by the views of stakeholders who were able to convincingly identify the benefits of the initiative at a local level. HAZs represent a useful recent example of a multi agency and multi faceted community-based health initiative. Evidence regarding their contribution, certainly in terms of that generated by the national evaluation, is perhaps best reviewed in conjunction with that produced from other complex initiatives of the same era. Results from other similar studies are now emerging, and a synthesis of evidence across this body of work would be useful in terms of generating policy lessons for health improvement efforts in the future.

References

Barnes, M., Sullivan, H. and Matka, E. (2003) Evidence, understanding and complexity: evaluation in non-linear systems, *Evaluation*, 9: 263–82.

Barnes, M., Bauld, L., Benzeval, M., Judge, K., Mackenzie, M. and Sullivan, H. (2005) *Health Action Zones: Partnerships for Health Equity*. London: Routledge.

Bauld, L., Judge, K., Lawson, L., Mackenzie, M., Mackinnon, J. and Truman, J. (2001) *Health Action Zones in Transition: Progress in 2000*. Glasgow: Health Promotion Policy Unit, University of Glasgow.

Bauld, L., Sullivan, H., Judge, K. and Mackinnon, J. (2005a) Assessing the impact of Health Action Zones, in M. Barnes *et al.* (eds) *Health Action Zones: Partnerships for Health Equity*. London: Routledge.

Bauld, L., Judge, K., Barnes, M., Benzeval, M., Mackenzie, M. and Sullivan, H. (2005b) Promoting social change: the experience of Health Action Zones in England, *Journal of Social Policy*, 34(3): 427–45.

Benzeval, M. (2005) Tackling health inequalities, in M. Barnes *et al.* (eds) *Health Action Zones: Partnerships for Health Equity*. London: Routledge.

Bertallanfy, L. von (1952) *General Systems Theory*. New York: Wiley.

Chapman, J. (2002) *System Failure: Why Governments must Learn to think Differently*. London: Demos.

Checkland, P. (1981) *Systems Thinking: Systems Practice*. New York: Wiley.

Checkland, P. and Scholes, J. (1990) *Soft Systems Methodology in Action*. Chichester: Wiley.

Connell, J.P., Kubisch, A.C., Schorr, L.B. and Weiss, C.H. (1995) *New Approaches to Evaluating Community Initiatives. Volume 1: Concepts, Methods and Contexts*. Washington, DC: The Aspen Institute.

Davies, H., Nutley, S. and Smith, P. (2000) *What Works: evidence based Policy and Practice in Public Services*. Bristol: Policy Press.

DoH (Department of Health) (1997) *Health Action Zones – Invitation to Bid*. Circular EL (97)65.

DoH (Department of Health) (1998a) Frank Dobson gives the go ahead for the first wave of Health Action Zones, press release 98/120. London: DoH.

DoH (Department of Health) (1998b) *Evaluation of Health Action Zones: Research Brief*. London: DoH Research and Development Division.

DoH (Department of Health) (1999) Seven million people to benefit from fifteen new Health Action Zones: further action taken to reduce health inequalities, press release 99/0259. London: DoH.

Fulbright-Anderson, K., Kubisch, A. and Connell, J. (eds) (1998) *New Approaches to Evaluating Community Initiatives. Volume 2: Theory, Measurement, and Analysis*. Washington, DC: The Aspen Institute.

Hebert, S. and Anderson, A. (1998) Applying the theory of change approach to two national, multisite comprehensive community initiatives, in K. Fulbright-Anderson, A. Kubisch and J. Connell (eds) *New Approaches to Evaluating Community Initiatives. Volume 2: Theory, Measurement, and Analysis*. Washington, DC: The Aspen Institute.

Judge, K. and Bauld, L. (2001) Strong theory, flexible methods: evaluating complex, community based initiatives, *Critical Public Health*, 11: 19–38.

Judge, K. and Bauld, L. (2006) Learning from policy failure? Health Action Zones in England, *European Journal of Public Health*, 16(4): 341–4.

Judge, K. and Mackenzie, M. (2002) Theory-based evaluation, in J. Machenback and M. Bakker (eds) *Reducing Inequalities in Health: A European Perspective*. London: Routledge.

Judge, K., Barnes, M., Bauld, L., Benzeval, M., Killoran, A., Robinson, R., Wigglesworth, R. and Zeilig, H. (1999) *Health Action Zones: Learning to Make a Difference*. Canterbury: PSSRU, University of Kent.

Killoran, A. and Popay, J. (2002) *Concepts and Methods: Stakeholders' Perspectives of Local Systems for Tackling Health Inequalities. An Exploratory Study*. London: Health Development Agency.

Mackenzie, M. and Benzeval, M. (2005) Evaluating policy and practice: designing the national HAZ evaluation, in M. Barnes *et al.* (eds) *Health Action Zones: Partnerships for Health Equity*. London: Routledge.

Mackenzie, M. and Blamey, A. (2005) The practice and the theory: lessons from the application of a theories of change approach, *Evaluation*, 11(2): 151–68.

Mackenzie, M., Lawson, L., Mackinnon, J. and Meth, F. (2005) Local strategies for whole systems change, in M. Barnes *et al.* (eds) *Health Action Zones: Partnerships for Health Equity*. London: Routledge.

Mackenzie, M., Blamey, A. and Hanlon, P. (2006) Using and generating evidence: policy makers' reflections on commissioning and learning from the Scottish Health Demonstration Projects, *Evidence and Policy*, 2(2): 211–26.

Martin, S. and Sanderson, I. (1999) Evaluating public policy experiments: measuring outcomes, monitoring processes or managing pilots? *Evaluation*, 5: 245–58.

Nutley, S., Walter, I. and Davies, H. (2003) From knowing to doing: a framework for understanding the evidence-into-practice agenda, *Evaluation,* 9: 125–48.

Pluye, P., Potvin, L. and Denis, J.-L. (2004) Making public health programs last: conceptualizing sustainability, *Evaluation and Program Planning,* 27: 121–33.

Pluye, P., Potvin, L., Denis, J.-L., Pelletier, J. and Mannoni, C. (2005) Program sustainability begins with the first events, *Evaluation and Program Planning,* 28: 123–37.

Sanderson, I. (2004) Getting evidence into practice: perspectives on rationality, *Evaluation,* 10(3): 366–79.

Stewart, M., Goss, S., Gillanders, G., Clarke, R., Rowe, J. and Shaftoe, H. (1999) *Cross-cutting Issues Affecting Local Government.* London: DETR.

Stewart, M., Gillanders, G., Goss, S., Grimshaw, L., Camerson, S. and Healy, P. (2002) *Collaboration and Co-ordination in Area-based Regeneration Initiatives: Final Report to the Department of Transport, Local Government and the Regions.* London: DETR.

Sullivan, H., Judge, K. and Sewel, K. (2004) 'In the eye of the beholder': perceptions of local impact in English Health Action Zones, *Social Science and Medicine,* 59(8): 1603–12.

Weiss, C.H. (1998) *Evaluation: Methods for Studying Programs and Policies,* 2nd edn. Englewood Cliffs, NJ: Prentice Hall.

Wilkinson, D. and Appelbee, E. (1999) *Implementing Holistic Government: Joined-up Action on the Ground.* Bristol: The Policy Press.

Young, K., Ashby, D., Boaz, A. and Grayson, L. (2002) Social science and the evidence based policy movement, *Social Policy and Society,* 1(3): 215–24.

13 Sure Start: an upstream approach to reducing health inequalities

Ben Gidley

Sure Start is a national initiative in the UK directed at preschool children and their families in disadvantaged areas. It seeks to develop improved and coordinated local services for families, enabling children to thrive as they enter school and on into later life. The Sure Start initiative was announced in 1997, very early in the first term of the New Labour government, and remains a central element in the government's strategy for social inclusion (Pugh 2003) (see also Chapter 6 and Chapter 14 for a full discussion on social inclusion).

The national Sure Start programme funds several local programmes, each based in deprived neighbourhoods. Local programmes are led by a variety of different lead agencies, including Primary Care Trusts, local authorities and voluntary sector agencies. Local programmes are given a great deal of freedom to develop different sorts of services and projects, depending on local needs and priorities. Core projects common to many local programmes include outreach and home visiting programmes; various support services for families and children; high-quality early childcare, learning and play opportunities; community healthcare, including information about child health and development; and support for children with special needs, such as special educational needs or speech and language issues (Melhuish *et al.* 2005).

This chapter will present Sure Start as an example of an upstream public health intervention. An upstream intervention is one that seeks to intervene in a social problem or a health problem early and deal with the causes rather than the symptoms. The development of upstream interventions is linked to what is called refocusing, a shift in balance from heavy-end provision, the treatment of the results of social or health problems (such as acute or restorative services), to front-end provision, which is prevention and early intervention before problems develop (Axford and Little 2005). Where heavy-end provision is costly, it has demonstrable results; front-end interventions might be cheaper in the long term, but they carry the risks of investment.

The term 'early' in the context of anticipatory intervention and prevention reflects not only an initial point in a problem's chain of causality, but also early in a person's life. There is a massive body evidence of the impact of early years on lifetime health. One such longitudinal study undertaken by Power *et al.* (1999), on a cohort of people born in 1958, found that disadvantage in infancy makes a contribution to the chances of poor health in adulthood, suggesting that long-term exposure to disadvantage is especially detrimental to health. Indeed, the weight of evidence suggests that a child's experiences in the early years are critical in shaping outcomes not just in health, but across education and welfare throughout that individual's lifespan (Hobcraft 1998; Bynner 2001; Davies and Wood 2002).

Consequently, early intervention in a child's life appears to be a wise investment. A number of early years interventions in recent decades have generated evidence of the efficacy of such upstream programmes to break the long-term effects of disadvantage (Hertzman 2000; Melhuish 2004; Axford and Little 2005). Two preschool programmes dating from the late 1960s and 1970s in the USA, Head Start and High/Scope, have particularly been the focus of scholarly research in this field (Lazar and Darlington 1982; Schweinhart *et al.* 1993; Schweinhart and Weikart 1997). Both these programmes were holistic, drawing on a range of professionals to intensively provide a range of services to families with children in their preschool years. Research using randomized trials found the programmes produced long-term benefits for participants, which led to significant public spending savings. Head Start was influential on the development of the Educational Priority Areas (EPAs) programme in the UK in the late 1960s, consisting of locally targeted interventions with strong preschool components in disadvantaged neighbourhoods. These interventions were also subject to robust evaluation using randomized control trials, which again contributed to the evidence for the efficacy of upstream interventions (Halsey 1972).

Sure Start, then, influenced by programmes like Head Start, was conceived as an upstream intervention in the sense that it explicitly set out to address the factors that give disadvantaged children a poor start in life. By intervening in these earliest years, it was assumed, the programme would be able to break what the New Labour government conceived as a cycle of disadvantage. The programme is central to a wider government objective to end child poverty, not simply as a good in itself, but as an upstream project of investment in the future.

In thinking about this sort of investment, and what it would take to break the cycle of disadvantage, it is important to distinguish upstream interventions from those policy instruments, such as reformed welfare, tax and tax credit systems, which seek to deal with the more structural factors that impact on poor families' health and wellbeing, such as lack of financial capital, a low wage economy, shelter poverty or social class more broadly. These structural factors are outside the power of a localized intervention like Sure Start, and may mark the limits of the efficacy of such a programme.

evidence based policy: a foundation for upstream intervention

There has been a strong trend in recent decades towards evidence based social policy instruments and a parallel utilitarian turn in the social sciences (Solesbury 2001). A strong evidence based tradition in medicine has spread to other areas, such as education, childcare and regeneration, where policy had previously reflected a more explicitly value- or ideology-led approach. Solesbury (2001) points to the post-1997 New Labour government's emphasis on a pragmatic or technocratic discourse of 'what works'. At the same time, there has been a greater recognition in the UK health sector from the late 1990s of the value of preventative medicine, particularly focusing on children and young people (see Chapter 2 for a historical context of public health and Chapter 11 for an examination of healthy public policies).

Consequently, a number of major initiatives have been put in place to capture more robust evidence of what does work in public health and children's health, such as evaluation research under the rubric of the Neighbourhood Renewal Unit, major evaluations of Health Action Zones (HAZs) (see Chapter 12) or the work of the National Institute of Clinical Excellence (NICE), all set up under the New Labour government. The national Sure Start programme had such an evidence based approach at its heart. Sure Start represents not only the most significant recent upstream intervention in early years health, but also the most significant attempt to systematically gather evidence of impact alongside delivery.

The design of the programme was based on attempts to collate evidence on what works. Norman Glass's Treasury-led Cross Departmental Review of Provision for Young Children, which created Sure Start, held seminars involving a wide range of experts and practitioners, to review the existing evidence on the factors involved in social exclusion risks in early childhood and their long-term consequences, and to review the evidence on the effectiveness of interventions directed at preschool children.

Not only was the design of the intervention heavily influenced by the available evidence, but the programme was intended to provide an even stronger evidence base for what works in early years interventions. In a sense, Sure Start was to provide a major laboratory for the study of such interventions. At a national level, an ambitious evaluation programme was designed into Sure Start. At a local level, programme design was required to reflect local needs analysis, and local programmes were required to conduct or commission regular local evaluations (Bynner *et al.* 1999).

Before the delivery of Sure Start began, an Evaluation Development Project was carried out to identify the best options for determining the effectiveness of Sure Start in meeting its aims (Bynner *et al.* 1999). There are broadly two types of evaluation: summative evaluation which seeks to draw conclusions about whether an intervention worked, and formative evaluation which is intended to contribute to the design or redesign of how an intervention is delivered (Kelly 2004). As the national Sure Start evaluation needed to both draw conclusions about the programme's efficacy and contribute to the ongoing development of Sure Start, both of these types of evaluation were integral. The Sure Start Evaluation Development Project used the terminology developed by the American Early Head Start programme, a recent early years focused element of the Head Start programme mentioned above, to distinguish between the research that would meet these two needs. An impact analysis would track the impact of Sure Start on its beneficiaries' lives into primary school achievements and achievements through secondary school and entry into adult life, comparing Sure Start areas in order to determine which features of the Sure Start programme proved most effective. An implementation analysis would investigate management and coordination, access to services, quantity and quality of services, allocation of resources and community involvement through a national survey, in-depth studies of 25 programmes and a series of themed evaluations. The aim was to use methods seen as scientifically robust to produce solid evidence, but to remain sensitive to local context. In addition, there was evaluation around cost-effectiveness, a cost–benefit analysis determining the efficacy of the spend on the programme, and support for local evaluations, training and other support to local programmes in commissioning and carrying out local evaluations (Melhuish and the National Evaluation of Sure Stare Team 1999).

Each local programme was expected to develop an evaluation framework and either implement the evaluation itself or, more commonly, commission independent evaluators. How this has worked in practice has varied enormously. In some cases, local programmes or clusters of local programmes developed ongoing partnerships with research teams to build evaluation into delivery (see for example Smith and Bryan 2005). In other cases, commissioning an evaluation was viewed as just one more burden imposed by the national Sure Start Unit, along with all the other monitoring programmes they were expected to carry out. For some, a more pragmatic approach was taken, with local programmes identifying specific research questions they were keen to answer. For example, one local programme commissioned an evaluation on why take-up of services appeared to be so high among black and minority ethnic families but so low among white families, while another commissioned an evaluation on how they might better work with male carers.

Local targeting, universalism and exclusion

A further key element in the Sure Start model is the principle of partnership. Although partnership was a central tenet of British regeneration policy under the Conservative governments of the 1980s, the New Labour policy instruments, such as the Single Regeneration Budget, have been characterized by an even stronger emphasis on partnerships. Based on the premise that successful interventions must be holistic, Sure Start seeks to work across institutional boundaries to secure the best outcomes. At the national level, this is reflected in the cross-departmental management of the Sure Start Unit. At the local level, it is reflected in the requirement for Sure Start programmes to be managed by partnership boards, with representation from a range of local stakeholders (Roberts 2000).

Local authorities and primary care authorities were expected to identify areas appropriate to the delivery of a Sure Start programme, based on indicators such as deprivation or low birth weights, and then bid competitively into the national Sure Start budget. Local programmes were to be based on local needs and priorities, some of which would be determined in advance of bidding, according to available quantitative indicators, while other needs and priorities would emerge through the life of the programme. Programmes carried out community needs assessments, ideally involving local communities in this process, and built in community engagement and evaluation mechanisms to ensure that other emerging needs would feed into delivery. This holistic area-based model strongly resonates with other social policy interventions of recent decades, such as Neighbourhood Renewal and the New Deal for Communities.

By definition, the areas targeted in area based initiatives have borders, which include some and exclude others. When funding is allocated to some areas and not others through competitive bidding, as with both Sure Start and its predecessors from City Challenge onwards, and when resources are scarce, the question of who is included and who is excluded can become politically contentious. Where neighbourhoods are divided from each other along real or imagined lines of race and ethnicity, this political contention can be particularly poisonous. For example, it is not uncommon in deprived areas, particularly in the inner city, for neighbourhoods perceived as, for example, white and areas perceived as Asian to be located adjacent to each other, because of histories of de facto segregation in the housing market or allocation policies, or because of accidents of settlement. If the Asian neighbourhood is given resources through Sure Start and not the white neighbourhood, or vice versa, a politics of competition can become a politics of resentment. This in turn can fuel white backlash far-right activity or the type of desperation that leads to urban violence, as in the Oldham riots of 2000 (Oldham Independent Review 2001).

The issue of who is included and who isn't has featured at a more personal level in a number of Sure Start evaluation projects, where workers complained of having to negotiate the ethical challenge of turning away or restricting users from outside the area, who may experience similar or even greater levels of need than users from within the target area.

Workers, because of Sure Start's distinctive ethos of universal provision, experience this ethical dilemma as acute. By defining a target population geographically, rather than on the basis of the needs or disadvantage of particular families, Sure Start ups the level of universal services within its area. There is, therefore, no stigma in being a Sure Start family in the way that there are stigmas associated with means-tested services, such as free school meals. This ethos of universal provision within a given area facilitates the possibility, which is not always realized, of Sure Start local programmes creating a sense of inclusion and ownership in the communities where they are located. Thus if anyone from a given neighbourhood with children under five has access to Sure Start services, then there is likely to be a stronger sense of ownership over the programme within that neighbourhood.

The corollary of this, however, is that socioeconomic grouping can become invisible in area-based interventions. If disadvantage is identified geographically, in terms of deprived neighbourhoods, then structures of poverty, and in particular cleavages of class, go out of focus. A frequent criticism of Sure Start, therefore, from users and workers and more frequently in the media (for example Colgan 2005; Bennett 2006) is that it provides free services for middle-class families. As deprived neighbourhoods are rarely universally deprived but often contain pockets of relative affluence, especially in inner cities and above all in inner London, less poor families can be entitled to Sure Start services by virtue of their address. Where they may already have a certain amount of resources or resourcefulness to take advantage more readily than some of their neighbours of opportunities offered by Sure Start, they may disproportionately access services they arguably need less.

A number of Sure Start projects were criticized along these lines by both parents and workers, most notably a post natal depression intervention using baby massage, and a literacy and numeracy focused play session. However, there are often more complex stories behind these perceptions. For example, interviewing mothers perceived by workers or other users as middle class, it was found that many were living in poverty, often as lone parents. Some parents from higher socioeconomic groups were also found to be not experiencing such a level of poverty, but experiencing severe isolation because of their dislocation from family or community networks, which is often more characteristic of working class culture.

However, a finding of the early evaluation report on Sure Start's impact is that Sure Start appears to be most beneficial for the relatively less disadvantaged families in disadvantaged areas, while there may actually be a negative effect on the most disadvantaged families, teenage parents, single parents and workless parents. The report conjectured that those with more resources to start with were able to access the higher level of services, possibly to the detriment of those who most needed them, a finding that also emerged with programmes such as Early Head Start in the USA (Melhuish *et al.* 2005; Belsky *et al.* 2006).

The focus on neighbourhoods in Sure Start is closely related to the communitarian political philosophy that has influenced New Labour social policy in the UK. This places an emphasis on community as the appropriate unit of intervention, and a localist ethos, which calls for devolution of decision making to the neighbourhood. There are two implications of the communitarian agenda behind Sure Start. The first is that local Sure Start programmes are enabled to develop very specific local styles and organizational cultures. The second is that, alongside the health focus of the programme, there is a strong community development dimension.

The communitarian, localist agenda behind Sure Start means that Sure Start local programmes grow very distinct local identities. Local programmes' needs assessments generate services and targets tailored to specific local needs; some local programmes might then focus on health issues, others on social issues, and so on. A vast array of partnership arrangements is possible within the national programme, so that very different organizational cultures prevail. For example, there are local programmes led by health service agencies, local authorities, voluntary-sector organizations and several different combinations of these. This might correspond to different sorts of venues where local programmes are based, from purpose-built centres and GP surgeries, to shop fronts and offices in council estate blocks. Each of these sends out a different sort of message to stakeholders.

All local programmes, however, are required to involve parents in management and decision making. The boards that manage programmes must comprise at least one-third parents and at least one-third community representatives. Programmes are expected to reach out to parents, to work with a community development ethos and, in particular, to engage the hard to reach. Programmes often employ parent involvement officers working alongside health and other professionals. The empowerment implied in this is viewed as a good in itself, but as also feeding into the upstream impact of the programme as empowerment is expected to contribute to a family's general wellbeing.

Governing families?

Sure Start's primary objectives are around supporting families, as part of an upstream initiative, including supporting families' participation in governing the way services are delivered locally. But critics have suggested that this emphasis on support is an attempt to regulate or govern the behaviour of families. Gillies and Edwards (2005) and Fawcett *et al.* (2004) argue that the intervention is premised on the assumption of the breakdown of the traditional family, with family conceived in an extremely conservative way, and predicated on an authoritarian intervention in parents' own behaviour and an increasing social control of childhood.

As already implied, at the heart of the Sure Start agenda is the concept of a cycle of disadvantage or deprivation. Gillies (2005a) traces the genealogy of this concept back to New Right thinking in the 1970s, which described deprivation as a *moral* problem passed on through poor families as part of a culture of dependency. In recent social policy discourse, the family is seen as the key space for producing what Nikolas Rose (1999, 2000) calls the liberal citizen. This is a citizen set free of the state, autonomous but required to act responsibly towards themselves and others – for example, eating healthily, not smoking, and parenting well, all key targets of Sure Start programmes.

Gillies (2005a) sees the New Labour emphasis on supporting families, as embodied in Sure Start, in this context. Sure Start offers material support for families in terms of access to high-quality childcare, but also moral support to do the right thing free of financial dependence on the state. Thus, support is conditional and implies a particular moral agenda that seeks to regulate and control the behaviour of marginalized families. Gillies argues that the normative model of successful parenting promoted by initiatives like Sure Start closely tallies with the values of white middle-class parents, which implicitly suggests that parents from other backgrounds by definition need intervention (Gillies 2005a). Gewirtz (2001) describes this as 'cloning the Blairs'. Similarly, Gillies sums up the New Labour view thus: 'For the sake of their children's future, and for the stability and security of society as a whole, working class parents must be taught how to raise middle class subjects' (2005b: 839).

For example, Sure Start's targets around getting mothers back into employment can be seen as part of a wider New Labour agenda around the moral imperative of productive work as an element of active citizenship (Vincent and Ball 2001; Osgood 2005), which can again be conceptualized in terms of Rose's figure of the liberal citizen. This emphasis on returning to work can also be tied back to the notion of social investment, upstream intervention in early years as a form of economic investment in the nation's future, with which this chapter began. Norman Glass, Sure Start's architect, has warned that the programme's initial child-centred focus is at risk because it is in danger of 'becoming a New Deal for toddlers', captured by the employability agenda (Lister 2006: 322).

Sure Start's legacy

The legacy of Sure Start is felt in a number of ways. A key successor intervention to Sure Start is the creation of Children's Centres. These are being introduced first in deprived neighbourhoods, with the intention of rolling them out nationally. They are premised on the Sure Start principles of multidisciplinary, inter-agency delivery, now embodied in a single location from which multiple services will be delivered. They build on a programme of Early Excellence Centres that ran parallel to Sure Start, which appear to have been successful in achieving similar outcomes to Sure Start, as well as cost savings (Bertram *et al.* 2002; Pugh 2002). Crucially, Children's Centres also build on the Sure Start principle of universal, and thus non stigmatizing, provision for a target area (Williams 2004). However, with their rolling out, there are significantly fewer resources available, and it remains to be seen whether the tighter budgets and wider spread will allow quality to be maintained.

The *Every Child Matters* Green Paper (Treasury Department 2003) set out a government commitment to generalize the upstream form of intervention that Sure Start has developed (Williams 2004). The core of *Every Child Matters* is a commitment to providing universal services for children that integrate targeted and specialist provision with a focus on early intervention and better prevention. Again, there is an emphasis on universalism and multidisciplinarity. In other words, *Every Child Matters* builds on all of the most positive aspects of Sure Start, widening its reach to the whole population, but with a lower level of resource.

As for Sure Start itself, in November 2005 the first report was published of the National Evaluation impact study (Melhuish *et al.* 2005). This concluded that there was little or no evidence of the beneficial impact of Sure Start. The media picked this up with gusto (Colgan 2005). However, the report itself was very clear that there is a massive difference between little or no evidence of impact and little or no actual impact.

There are a number of factors making it hard to judge whether Sure Start has had its intended impact as an upstream intervention. First, simply, it is too early. It can take three years for a local programme to fully get off the ground (Melhuish *et al.* 2005), and the impacts on a child's life will emerge slowly over the years as they start school. Second, there are issues of sampling that make it hard to review the evidence. Randomized control trials, for example, were simply not possible with an intervention of such complexity. Third, local Sure Start local programmes are so varied that it can be difficult to compare them with each other and with the matched areas.

Fourth, and key, is the fact that Sure Start is being delivered alongside a plethora of other initiatives, which are also being delivered in the comparison areas. For example, one of the Sure Start areas we evaluated was also a Single Regeneration Budget area, a Neighbourhood Management area, an Education Action Zone area and part of an HAZ area (see Chapter 12 for further discussion of HAZs). Other complicating factors in this area included periodic reorganizations of the National Health Service (NHS), the transfer of housing stock from the local authority to a different social landlord, the influx of residents from other areas of the borough being decanted due to physical regeneration schemes on other estates, a community anti-racist initiative, and the construction of a new leisure centre. Given this multiplicity, disaggregating what Sure Start caused from what was caused by other initiatives is impossible.

Nonetheless, there is evidence that Sure Start has had a positive impact. Prior to Sure Start, the provision of early years services was characterized by a lack of strategy and joined up thinking, with a multiplicity of providers across sectors delivering uneven services that varied greatly from place to place, but this diversity did not mean choice for parents. There were low levels of public funding and a reliance on the voluntary and private sectors (Pugh 1996). Sure Start has exemplified a fundamental break with this state of affairs. Services are clearly designed according to a more holistic and strategic framework; professionals work outside their disciplines, sharing data and jointly implanting strategies. Delivery is joined up across sectors rather than ad hoc and patchy, and it is the most deprived areas that have benefited from this. In particular, Sure Start indicates a recognition that care for children is a public good and not simply a private duty.

References

Axford, N. and Little, M. (2005) Refocusing children's services towards prevention: lessons from the literature, *Children and Society*, 20: 299–312.

Belsky, J., Melhuish, E., Barnes, J., Leyland, A., Romaniuk, H. and the NESS Research Team (2006) Effects of Sure Start local programmes on children and families: early findings from a quasi-experimental, cross sectional study, *British Medical Journal*, 7556: 1476–9.

Bennett, R. (2006) Poor turned off Sure Start by middle-class mothers, *The Times*, 6 October.

Bertram, T., Pascal, C., Bokhari, S., Gasper, M. and Holtermanm, S. (2002) *Early Excellence Centre Pilot Programme: Second Evaluation Report 2000–2001*. London: DfES.

Bynner, J. (2001) Childhood risks and protective factors in social exclusion, *Children and Society*, 15: 285–301.

Bynner, J., Ferri, E., Plewis, I., Kelly, Y., Marmot, M., Pickering, K., Smith, T. and Smith, G. (1999) *Sure Start Evaluation Development Project: Report to Sure Start Unit*. London: Sure Start Evaluation Development Project.

Colgan, J. (2005) View from a broad, *Guardian*, 2 December.

Davies, E. and Wood, B. (2002) From rhetoric to action: a case for a comprehensive community based initiative to improve developmental outcomes for disadvantaged children, *Social Policy Journal of New Zealand*, 19: 28–47.

Fawcett, B., Featherstone, B. and Goddard, J. (2004) *Contemporary Child Care Policy and Practice*. Basingstoke: Palgrave Macmillan.

Gewirtz, S. (2001) Cloning the Blairs: New Labour's programme for the re-socialization of working class parents, *Journal of Education Policy*, 16: 365–78.

Gillies, V. (2005a) Meeting parents' needs? Discourses of 'support' and 'inclusion' in family policy, *Critical Social Policy*, 25: 70–90.

Gillies, V. (2005b) Raising the 'meritocracy': parenting and the individualisation of social class, *Sociology*, 39: 835–53.

Gillies, V. and Edwards, R. (2005) Secondary analysis in exploring family and social change: addressing the issue of context, *Forum: Qualitative Social Research*, 6: 44.

Halsey, A. (1972) *EPA: Problems and Policies, Educational Priority*, Volume 1. London: HMSO.

Hertzman, C. (2000) The case for an early childhood strategy, *Isuma*, 1(2): 11–18.

Hobcraft, J. (1998) *Intergenerational and Life Course Transmission of Social Exclusion: Influences of Childhood Poverty, Family Disruption and Contact with the Police*. London: Centre for Analysis of Social Exclusion.

Kelly, M. (2004) Qualitative evaluation research, in C. Seale *et al.* (eds) *Qualitative Research Practice*. London: Sage.

Lazar, I. and Darlington, R. (1982) *Lasting Effects of Early Education: A Report from the Consortium for Longitudinal Studies*. London: Society for Research in Child Development.

Lister, R. (2006) Children (but not women) first: New Labour, child welfare and gender, *Critical Social Policy*, 26: 315–35.

Melhuish, E.C. (2004) *A Literature Review of the Impact of Early Years Provision on Young Children, with Emphasis Given to Children from Disadvantaged Backgrounds*. London: Institute for the Study of Children, Families and Social Issues.

Melhuish, E.C. and the National Evaluation of Sure Start Team (1999) *National Evaluation of Sure Start: Summary*. London: Sure Start.

Melhuish, E., Belsky, J. and Leyland, A. (2005) *Early Impacts of Sure Start Local Programmes on Children and Families: Report of the Cross-sectional Study of 9 and 36 Month Old Children and their Families*. London: HMSO.

Oldham Independent Review (2001) *Panel Report*. Oldham: Oldham Independent Review.

Osgood, J. (2005) Who cares? The classed nature of childcare, *Gender and Education*, 17: 289–303.

Power, C., Manor, O. and Matthews, S. (1999) The duration and timing of exposure: effects of socioeconomic environment on adult health, *American Journal of Public Health*, 89: 1059–65.

Pugh, G. (ed.) (1996) *Contemporary Issues in the Early Years: Working Collaboratively for Children*, 2nd edn. London: Paul Chapman.

Pugh, G. (2002) Services fit for young children and their families? in K. White (ed.) *Re-framing Children's Services*. London: NCVCCO.

Pugh, G. (2003) Early childhood services: evolution or revolution? *Children & Society*, 17: 184–94.

Roberts, H. (2000) What is Sure Start? *Archives of Disease in Childhood*, 82: 435–7.

Rose, N. (1999) *Powers of Freedom: Reframing Political Thought*. Cambridge: Cambridge University Press.

Rose, N. (2000) Community, citizenship and the Third Way, *American Behaviour Scientist*, 43: 1395–411.

Schweinhart, L.J. and Weikart, D.P. (1997) *Lasting Differences: The High/Scope Preschool Curriculum Comparison Study Through Age 27*. Ypsilanti, MI: The High/Scope Press.

Schweinhart, L.J., Barnes, H.V. and Weikart, D.P. (1993) *Significant Benefits: The High/Scope Perry Preschool Study Through Age 23*. Ypsilanti, MI: The High/Scope Press.

Smith, P. and Bryan, K. (2005) Participatory evaluation: navigating the emotions of partnerships, *Journal of Social Work Practice*, 19: 195–209.

Solesbury, W. (2001) *Evidence Based Policy: Whence it Came and Where it's Going*. London: ESRC UK Centre for Evidence Based Policy and Practice.

Treasury Department (2003) *Every Child Matters*. London: The Stationery Office.

Vincent, C. and Ball, S. (2001) A market in love? Choosing pre-school childcare, *British Educational Research Journal*, 27: 633–51.

Williams, F. (2004) What matters is who works: why every child matters to New Labour. Commentary on the DfES Green Paper *Every Child Matters*, *Critical Social Policy*, 24: 406–27.

14 Community participation for health: reducing health inequalities and building social capital

Antony Morgan and Jennie Popay

Involving communities of place and/or interest in all aspects of the development, implementation and evaluation of health development and social regeneration programmes has become commonplace and is now an explicit requirement of many government strategies to tackle health inequalities (WHO 1999; DoH 2004).

The primary purpose of engaging communities from a policy perspective is to promote more responsive public services, to help improve quality and to support civic renewal (Hamer 2005). Put another way, community engagement is regarded as having the potential to improve the quality of the service supplied and the opportunities and capacities of those who rely on services (Rogers and Robinson 2004).

However, despite the commitment to community level action in policy terms, at least at the rhetorical level, the practice of how to do it effectively has proved highly complex. Pickin (2002) identifies several important reasons for ensuring that appropriate and effective involvement is achieved. First, without involvement, access cannot be gained to the resources, assets, skills and first hand knowledge of local people and service users. Second, without this access, policies and services are less likely to be appropriate to need and to be owned by the people they are aimed at. Third, if policies and services are seen as inappropriate and not owned by the people they are aimed at, they will be less likely to be effective, and innovation will be unsustainable.

The purpose of this chapter is to summarize the findings from the Social Action for Health programme (Pickin 2002; Swann and Morgan 2002; Morgan and Swann 2005), which aimed to establish a firmer evidence base for the benefits of participative approaches to reducing health inequalities using the concept of social capital as a framework for action. In particular the chapter focuses on the findings from a social action research project which sought to understand the conditions required for effective community involvement. In doing so it highlights a number of issues that need to be addressed by national and local government and professionals in public health and other sectors if well-intentioned policies and initiatives seeking to tackle health inequalities are to be successful.

Community participation and social models for health

Globally, public health agendas have recognized that health experience is shaped by genetic factors, individual lifestyles and a wide range of social, cultural, economic, political and environmental factors (Davey 2005; Garman 2005; McDaid and Oliver 2005; Scriven 2005). Over the last 25 years these agendas have been driven and developed by a growing body of evidence that demonstrates that those who live in disadvantaged social circumstances have more illness, greater distress, more disability and shorter lives than those who are more affluent (Dahlgren and Whitehead 1992; Townsend *et al.* 1992; Acheson 1998; Mackenbach and Bakker 2002; Wilkinson 2005, and Chapters 3 and 4 of this text). Explanations about the causes of inequalities in health are complex. Structural factors such as physical circumstances and material capital have been identified as having a key role. Conditions of poor housing and sanitation (see Chapter 18), poverty and inadequate diet from lack of income all contribute to poor health.

However, the existence of a gradient even among the Whitehall cohort of relatively advantaged civil servants indicates that factors additional to absolute poverty contribute to inequalities (Marmot *et al.* 1991). Wilkinson has shown that the degree of economic inequality within a society is related to increased mortality at a population level. He argues that the effects of inequality manifest themselves through the mechanisms of decreasing social cohesion that result in increased poor health among members of that society. Equitable societies with strong social support and social cohesion have better health outcomes (Wilkinson 2005). Wilkinson (2000) has also argued that there are very important psychosocial pathways through which people's circumstances affect their health and that social affiliations and friendship networks appear to be highly protective of health. It is clear then that a combination of factors is at work, reflecting people's living and working conditions, their resources, social relationships and lifestyles.

Building evidence for effective action on inequalities

Despite the momentum at policy level, the current state of evidence about interventions that might work to achieve the objective of reducing inequalities in health is limited. While there is a growing acknowledgement of the relationship between poverty and poor health outcomes, far less is known about how to challenge and change health inequalities (Gillies 1998; Exworthy and Powell 2000). Indeed, we are rich in data about the extent of the inequalities that exist, but we know much less about how most effectively to intervene to do something about them (Millard 2001). Nonetheless recent national and international initiatives (Acheson 1998; International Union of Health Promotion and Education 2000; Mackenbach and Bakker 2002), have attempted to understand the precise nature of the causal pathways and the different dimensions of inequality, the implications of demographic changes and their differential effects by social groupings, and the ways in which interventions work in different segments of the population.

These initiatives suggest that key characteristics of successful equity focused policies would involve a combination of approaches and methods that promote:

- regeneration through social and economic development;
- integrated packages of services provided by health and local authorities responding to the specific needs of individuals and families;
- community development initiatives and projects concerned particularly with engaging lay communities in decisions affecting their lives and developing the capability of communities and of public-sector organizations in health promotion practice, and addressing the wider factors that impact on their health.

Given the commitment to participation in policy development and implementation, the issue of evidence and community based action is increasingly important for strategists, policy makers and practitioners. This commitment can be sustained only if area based initiatives aiming to promote community action can produce demonstrable or measurable changes in health and/or its underlying determinants. However, the development of an evidence base in this area is fraught with challenges not least because of the long-term changes that community based activity produce and the associated difficulties in ascertaining causality with longer-term outcomes. When evaluation attempts have been made, they are often conducted over too short a time frame to identify long, term outcomes (Popay 2006), leaving many unconvinced of the return on investment. Building a credible evidence base for effective action in this area will be achieved only if policy makers accept the range of intermediate outcomes, such as increased social capital, including neighbourhood participation, increased sense of empowerment and the improved communication between communities and service providers that can be achieved in the short to medium term. Demonstration of the longer-term impacts of community approaches, such as the effect on mortality and/or morbidity rates, can be made only if adequate investment is made in appropriate types of evaluation methods and techniques over a meaningful time frame.

In the meantime, there is a need to understand how to most effectively engage the public in all aspects of the health development process. Existing evidence (NHS Centre for Reviews and Dissemination 1997) highlights the key characteristics of successful social approaches as including:

- local assessment of needs, especially involving local people in the research process itself;
- mechanisms that enable organizations to work together, ensuring dialogue, contact and commitment;
- representation of local people within planning and management arrangements. The greater the level of involvement, the larger the impact;
- design of specific initiatives with target groups to ensure that they are acceptable culturally and are educationally appropriate, and that they work through settings that are accessible and appropriate;
- training and support for volunteers, peer educators and local networks, thus ensuring maximum benefit from community based initiatives;
- visibility of political support and commitment;
- reorientation of resource allocation to enable systematic investment in community based programmes;

- policy development and implementation that brings about wider changes in organizational priorities and policies, driven by community based approaches;
- increased flexibility of organizations, so supporting increased delegation and a more responsive approach.

Social Action for Health sought to build on this existing evidence base by exploring the concept of social capital and its potential (Gillies 1998; Baum 2000) for using community and civic pathways to promote and improve health and tackle inequalities in health. Social capital is a multi component concept comprising indicators that attempt to measure the range of social relationships and networks both formal and informal that individuals and communities might possess which are health promoting (see Chapter 6 for a detailed examination of social capital).

Gillies (1998) claims that social capital can make a contribution to the reduction in inequalities in at least two ways. First, it revitalizes the debate and discussion about the importance of social approaches to public health and health promotion and, second, although not yet a theory with explanatory power, social capital allows us to examine the processes whereby social connections operating through a range of different types of networks can act as a buffer against the worst effects of deprivation. In doing so it offers a new package of social indicators for measuring community based interventions for health.

Social capital and the inequalities agenda

The idea of social capital has become increasingly prominent in international and national policy making as one potential concept that may contribute to the further understanding of the social determinants of health. It is a hotly disputed concept, but has been put forward by some authors (Gillies 1998; Campbell *et al.* 1999) as a potential explanation of how community-level factors may influence health and act as a buffer against the worst effects of poverty and deprivation. Campbell *et al.* (1999) promote social capital as a useful tool to help us understand the extent to which community-level relationships and networks might impact on health in local communities.

Various authors have depicted social capital as a mediating link between socio-economic inequality and health. In particular Wilkinson (2005) argues that socio-economic inequality affects health because it erodes social capital. Campbell *et al.* (1999) suggest that social capital can act as a buffer against socio economic disadvantage by reducing the effects of the lack of economic resources, and Cooper *et al.* (1999) have demonstrated a modest independent effect of some indicators of social capital on health after controlling for a range of socioeconomic variables.

Social capital has been defined in many ways based on different theoretical perspectives (Bourdieu 1986; Coleman 1988; Putnam 1993b), however common to all these definitions is that social capital is a resource for societies. It is essentially about networks of different types, shapes and sizes. Communities where social capital is abundant are often characterized by high levels of trust between friends and neighbours, shared norms and values, and local people actively engaged in civic and community life (Campbell *et al.* 1999; Morgan and Swann 2005).

Some authors purport that social capital is an old idea with a new name. Lynch *et al.* (2000), for example, argue that such under theorized applications in health research have led to social capital being applied as a new and more fashionable label for investigations that used to be called social support. Others (Portes and Landolt 1996) warn that social capital has its dark sides potentially promoting strong community ties, which sometimes result in the exclusion of outsiders (across ethnic groups for example) and restrictions on individual freedoms. Portes also believes that some governments may use social capital as an excuse not to act on the structural determinants of health, such as creating job opportunities.

Different forms of social capital have been identified (Woolcock 2001; Aldridge and Halpern 2002):

- *bonding social capital*, characterized by strong bonds, or social glue, within groups, such as among family members or members of an ethnic group;
- *bridging social capital*, characterised by weaker, less dense but more cross-cutting ties, or social oil, such as business associations or friends from different ethnic groups;
- *linking social capital*, characterized by connections between differing levels of power or social status, such as links between the political elite and the general public or between individuals from different social classes.

What are the links to health?

Existing research has shown that increasing social capital in local communities can result in reductions in infant mortality and increased life expectancy (Putnam 1993b), improved survival from heart disease and lower death rates from stroke, accidents and suicide. Social Action for Health gave further support to this evidence. Cooper *et al.* (1999) for example, found that social capital and social support were related to an individual's age, gender, socioeconomic circumstances and material living conditions, and that it is essential that surveys collect information about all these variables and examine the contribution of social capital and social support to health and health-related behaviour after adjusting for these structural factors. In addition, Pevalin and Rose (2003) found that all measures of social capital and social support except contact with friends reduced the likelihood of common mental illness and poor self-rated health.

However Social Action for Health also concluded that while some independent effects have been found, social capital has less power to predict health than other more familiar indicators of socioeconomic status. Moreover, the programme found different patterns of association between different indicators of social capital and different health outcomes (Ginn and Arber 2004; Pevalin 2004). It called for further empirical research to employ a detailed taxonomy that explicitly frames the concept and all its component parts, as well as the range of outcomes that might benefit from investments in it. Such a taxonomy will allow systematic empirical testing of the concept against a range of hypotheses that seek to unravel the mechanisms through which social capital operates to develop health and reduce health inequalities.

Overall, while social capital should not be seen as an alternative to changing the structural drivers of inequality, Gillies (1998) argues that low levels of social capital can undermine the effectiveness of community based initiatives.

Two important elements of community based approaches to health improvement which governments promote in public health strategies aiming to tackle health inequalities are the use of participatory approaches in health promotion and public health and the engagement of individuals in social networks.

These are also crucial elements of social capital, and it thus provides a framework for measuring the effectiveness of community based approaches to health improvement and inequalities. It does this by identifying indicators that can:

- assess the extent to which local people can participate in all aspects of the planning, development and evaluation of initiatives;
- describe the mechanisms required to ensure organizations work effectively together in ways that cross professional and lay boundaries;
- measure the amount and type of formal and informal outward looking social and civic networks that have been developed which can support better access to services and information.

Engaging local communities, building social capital

The Social Action for Health programme set up demonstration sites that used action research to test a range of methods for stimulating social action in neighbourhoods, working on the basis that increased social interaction would generate a stronger sense of community, more reciprocal relationships and a greater commitment to place, and hence have an impact on people's health. It sought to develop our understanding of the importance of multi sectoral partnerships including lay people as equal but different partners around the table and the democratization of decision making, and their relationship to health improvement.

The Salford Social Action Research Project (SARP) was set up as part of the programme to identify ways of connecting people living in neighbourhoods that were experiencing extreme social and economic disadvantage and in which services were of poor quality and/or inaccessible for a range of reasons, and support them to engage in social action for change and improvement. It used the indicators of social capital to evaluate its work and sought to develop practice by experimenting with ways of developing and sustaining various forms of social capital within localities experiencing significant disadvantage. In particular it focused on activities associated with linking social capital to promote more effective relationships between local people and public-sector organizations. There was an explicit attempt to focus on the development of capacity for social action within lay communities and the development of capacity for working equality with lay people within the public-sector agencies that served these communities.

The Salford SARP project was unlike many other *policy initiatives* in a number of ways.

- Its programme of activities were not elaborated against defined policy targets. This gave it the freedom to devise a range of actions based on a set of principles (including effective research and policy dialogue, social agitation and innovation), but be firmly led by the needs of the community rather than the priorities identified by policy makers.

- Local people were employed, eventually by the university due to process difficulties with other public agencies, as social action coordinators in local areas. These were key personnel in the model of change with the role of promoting active involvement of members of their communities.
- The use of participative, inclusive approaches to community planning, decision making and collective action, and the creation of space for learning and innovative thinking about existing practices and community involvement.
- The provision of sophisticated capacity building support for local people, akin to the high-quality organizational development support that many public agencies buy in to resource community groups appropriately for their partnership work with public-sector agencies. This was an explicit attempt to shift the balance of power in relationships between local people and public-sector agencies and professionals.

What did SARP do differently?

SARP action at neighbourhood level was initiated by each of four local action co-ordinators appointed by SARP to get people involved in long-term community action in their area to improve quality of life. The local action coordinators had personalized support from professional facilitators who helped them to decide on how to elucidate local issues and how to plan and implement action to address these issues. Through this process SARP identified local significant issues and a process or method by which a suitable set of interested parties, bridging community and local agencies, could be brought together to consider the issues and how to address them in partnership.

It differed from many other community based initiatives in the following ways.

- *Shifting the focus from individuals to collective social action.* SARP combined the strengths of individual social agitators with those of collective social action. Local action coordinators were employed and trained to encourage and support collective action among local residents rather than increasing their capacity to take action in their own right. This approach widened the pool of local people who were willing and able to take part in action aiming to improve life in the local neighbourhoods. In this way, purposeful, selective and committed involvement rather than representation was achieved.
- *Putting organizational change before community capacity.* Public organizations, despite emphasis in public strategies, often do not see involvement as integral to their work, resulting in tokenistic and poor-quality involvement. Involving communities in a meaningful way is often seen as coupled with a loss of control, leading to a breakdown in trust between organizations and local communities. There is a perceived tension between involving the lay public and responding to the pressures of upward accountability.
- *Making use of information and communication technology to promote innovation in engagement.* One example used by SARP involved the use of virtual reality

technology to translate housing demolition and restructuring proposals into 3D virtual streets, allowing local residents to see and experience what their area would look like after demolition and remodelling of existing houses. Residents identified problems with the proposals, leading to a complete reworking of the original plans with much greater involvement of local people.

- *Methods for working whole systems.* SARP set out to specifically support collective deliberation in ways that would lead to voice, dialogue and action and signal a more equal partnership between communities and public agencies. This led to a view that the methods for involvement needed to be varied and capable of responding to specific conditions and circumstances, and supportive of deliberative practice. Some of SARP invested in a number of facilitative or enabling technologies including: whole systems working and other interactive, participative methods such as mediation and large group methods; participatory appraisal; action learning; social and economic technologies such as time banking; community arts and information technology based systems. The methods performed different combinations of function: Combining facilitators and techniques to orchestrate and foster linkage and exchange between participants and so promoting forms of bonding, bridging and linkage; articulation and expression in which issues could be debated and defined; expressing and strengthening shared identity and belonging within communities; a means of reaching decisions and committing to action. The use of deliberative approaches to engagement resulted in the development of a more prepositional base for community involvement in regeneration planning. This represented a move away from institutionally mandated authorities following prescribed procedures for accomplishing goals, as is common in many area based policy initiatives.

- *Moving from capacity building to capacity release.* Historically there has been a view that the lay public in poor areas do not have the capacity to become involved in developing and carrying out policy, or in the governance of community affairs. SARP sought ways of moving away from this deficit model towards an asset-based model of community appraisal (Kretzmann and McKnight 1993), which encouraged a focus on community assets and not just on needs. Once the assets of communities have been identified, work can then take place to remove the barriers to releasing the capacity these assets represent.

- *Moving from skills training to shared learning.* Action coordinators took risks as they sought to understand the perspective of public-sector organizations and to work constructively with them; public service workers took risks through opening up their work to scrutiny and challenge by local communities. All organizations took risks in trying to communicate honestly and openly with partner agencies and members of the public about current difficulties and past mistakes. Risk-taking individuals and organizations can be sustained only in a shared learning environment that creates a climate in which effective learning is a crucial goal and activity.

- *Shifting the focus from resources to community resourcefulness.* SARP found that people living in very disadvantaged areas have a wide range of resources to bring to bear on the problems they face. SARP therefore developed ways in which these resources could be used to maximum effect, to improve the social and material conditions of local people in collaboration with public service organizations. Cognitive mapping was used to reveal in a visual way people's views, opinions and assumptions, and their theories about a given issue. Merging of maps showed where beliefs about an issue were shared among different participants and where they differed.

What did SARP reveal about community involvement?

Those involved with SARP and its evaluation were able to ascertain the impact on community involvement (Ford 2000; Popay and Finnegan 2005). SARP promoted community engagement as an end in itself rather than a means to an end. It was not a mechanism for delivering somebody else's agenda but rather a means for ensuring that the community's agenda was taken seriously and acted on. There is evidence that SARP's intervention did contribute to the delivery of policy targets but this was an indirect benefit of the engagement process. SARP successfully sought to avoid either becoming a part of the system of delivery or remaining outside the mainstream. Rather it sought to complement, challenge and support delivery organizations. It did so by:

- developing and supporting equal partnerships between lay publics and senior policy makers in public agencies with a primary focus on shared learning rather than policy implementation;
- acknowledging a strictly limited life from the outset;
- seeking to spark and support innovations in practice consistent with its principles;
- maintaining a strong culture of learning;
- challenging and aiming high where a principle and direction of change in practice was involved.

Effective community involvement was achieved by:

- creating conditions which allowed connections within and between communities to be made, acknowledging and working with tensions and conflicts within communities;
- challenging the conduct and assumptions of public sector agencies and workers at all levels and supporting the development of shared learning between the lay and professional worlds, contributing to better quality relationships between community and public organizations;
- having the flexibility to bring resources to bear on problems through the use of innovative approaches including deliberative approaches and formal mediation;
- employing appropriate professional experts who understood the science of building partnerships, and community experts who were skilled in encouraging and supporting collective action in their communities on burning issues;
- offering the communities a fundamentally different deal – SARP communities were given the freedom to create an emergent local agenda of shared purpose, built with the permission and active support of local agencies.

Importantly, from the outset SARP was driven by a critical mass of senior managers and politicians with a shared commitment to the principles and practices of effective community governance, willing and able to support action on significant issues for local communities and to promote radically different ways of thinking about community and public-sector partnerships. In this way SARP had a significant impact on the development of social relationships within and between communities and between communities and the public agencies there to serve them, arguably the conditions that are required to build social capital within and between lay communities and organizations.

Commitment by policy makers to involve local communities in the process of health development is not in itself enough to make it happen. Effective community engagement is dependent on the implementation of initiatives that seek to release the considerable capacity for action that exists within both lay communities and organizations.

SARP found that a combination of impassioned local people, policy makers and service providers willing to take risks made it much more likely that effective partnerships between the lay public, policy makers and service providers would emerge.

Thus SARP has found that public involvement policies need to give due weight to building the capacity of people in public service organizations to engage in more participatory and equal relationships with local populations. They need to be encouraged to take the expertise and experience of the lay communities they work with more seriously, to recognize that without this expertise and experience effective action to reduce health inequalities is neither possible nor sustainable.

References

Acheson, D. (1998) *Independent Inquiry into Inequalities in Health – Report*. London: The Stationery Office.

Aldridge, S. and Halpern, D. (2002) *Social Capital: A Discussion Paper*. London: The Cabinet Office, Performance and Innovation Unit.

Baum, F. (2000) Social capital, economic capital and power: further issues for a public health agenda, *Journal of Epidemiology Community Health*, 54: 409–10.

Bourdieu, P. (1986) The forms of capital, in J. Richardson (ed.) *Handbook of Theory and Research for the Sociology of Education*. New York: Macmillan.

Campbell, C., Wood, R. and Kelly, M. (1999) *Social Capital and Health*. London: Health Education Authority.

Coleman, J. (1988) Social capital in the creation of human capital, *American Journal of Sociology*, 94 (supplement): S95–120.

Cooper, H., Arber, S., Fee, L. and Ginn, J. (1999) *The Influence of Social Support and Social Capital for Health*. London: Health Education Authority.

Dahlgren, G. and Whitehead, M. (1992) *Policies and Strategies to Promote Equity in Health*. Copenhagen: WHO Regional Office for Europe.

Davey, B. (2005) Key global heath concerns in the 21st century, in A. Scriven and S. Garman (eds) *Promoting Health: Global Perspectives*. Basingstoke: Palgrave Macmillan.

DoH (Department of Health) (2004) *Choosing Health: Making Healthier Choices Easier*. London: the Stationery Office.

Exworthy, M. and Powell, M.A. (2000) *Understanding Health Variations and Policy Variations*. Lancaster: Economic and Social Research Council (Research Findings 5).

Ford, K. (2000) *A Report of the HEA's Social Action Research Project Network Meeting*. London: Health Education Authority.

Garman, S. (2005) The social context of health promotion in a globalising world, in A. Scriven and S. Garman (eds) *Promoting Health: Global Perspectives*. Basingstoke: Palgrave Macmillan.

Gillies, P. (1998) The effectiveness of alliances and partnerships for health promotion, *Health Promotion International,* 13(2): 99–120.

Ginn, J. and Arber, S. (2004) Gender and the relationship between social capital and health, in A. Morgan and C. Swann (eds) *Social Capital and Health: Issues of Definition, Measurement and Links to Health*. London: Health Development Agency.

Hamer, L. (2005) *Community Engagement for Health: A Preliminary Review of Training and Development Needs and Existing Provision for Public Sector Organisations and their Workers*. London: NICE.

International Union of Health Promotion and Education (2000*) The Evidence of Health Promotion Effectiveness: Shaping Public Health in Europe. A Report for the European Commission by the International Union for Health Promotion and Education*. Brussels and Luxembourg: International Union for Health Promotion and Education.

Kretzmann, J.P. and McKnight, J.L. (1993) *Building Communities from the Inside Out: a Path Toward Finding and Mobilizing a Community's Assets*. Evanston, IL: The Asset-Based Community Development Institute, Institute for Policy Research.

Lynch, J., Due, P. and Mutaneer, C. (2000) Social capital – it is a good investment strategy for public health, *Journal of Epidemiology Community Health*, 54: 404–8.

Mackenbach, J. and Bakker, M. (eds) (2002) *Reducing Inequalities in Health: A European Perspective*. London: Routledge.

McDaid, D. and Oliver, A. (2005) Inequalities in health: international patterns and trends, in: A. Scriven and S. Garman (eds) *Promoting Health: Global Perspectives*. Basingstoke: Palgrave Macmillan.

Marmot, M.G., Davey-Smith, G., Stansfield, S., Patel, C., North, F., Head, J., White, I., Brunner, E. and Feeney, A. (1991) Health inequalities among British civil servants: the Whitehall II study, *The Lancet*, 337: 1387–93.

Millard, L. (2001) *Public Health Intervention Research – The Evidence*. London: Health Development Agency.

Morgan, A. and Swann, C. (2005) *Social Capital and Health: Issues of Definition, Measurement and Links to Health*. London: Health Development Agency.

NHS Centre for Reviews and Dissemination (1997) *Review of Effectiveness of Interventions Aimed at Reducing Inequalities in Health*. York: University of York.

Pevalin, D.J. (2004) Intra-household differences in neighbourhood attachment and their associations with health, in A. Morgan and C. Swann (eds) *Social Capital and Health: Issues of Definition, Measurement and Links to Health*. London: Health Development Agency.

Pevalin, D.J. and Rose, D. (2003) *Social Capital for Health: Investigating the Links Between Social Capital and Health Using the British Household Panel Survey*. London: Health Development Agency.

Pickin, C. (2002) *Involving Lay Publics in Developing Policy and Services*. London: Health Development Agency.

Popay, J. (2006) *Community Engagement for Health Improvement: Questions of Definition Outcomes and Evaluation*. A background paper prepared for NICE.

Popay, J. and Finnegan, H. (2005) *Learning About Effective Community Engagement from Selected National Initiatives*. Lancaster: National Collaborating Centre, Lancaster University, working paper 5.

Portes, A. and Landolt, P. (1996) The downside of social capital, *The American Prospect,* 26: 18–21.

Putnam, R. (1993a) The prosperous community: social capital and public life, *The American Prospect,* 13: 1–8.

Putnam, R. (1993b). *Making Democracy Work: Civic Traditions in Modern Italy*. Princeton, NJ: Princeton University Press.

Rogers, B. and Robinson, E. (2004) *Active Citizenship Centre Report – The Benefits of Community Engagement: A Review of the Evidence*. London: Institute of Public Policy Research.

Scriven, A. (2005) Promoting health: a global context and rationale, in A. Scriven and S. Garman (eds) *Promoting Health: Global Perspectives*. Basingstoke: Palgrave Macmillan.

Swann, C. and Morgan, A. (eds) (2002) *Social Capital for Health: Insights from Qualitative Research*. London: Health Development Agency.

Townsend, P., Davidson, N. and Whitehead, M. (1992) *Inequalities in Health: The Black Report and the Health Divide*. London: Penguin.

WHO (World Health Organization) (1999) *Health 21: The Health for All Policy Framework for the WHO European Region*. Copenhagen: WHO Regional Office for Europe.

Wilkinson, R.G. (2000) Inequality and the social environment: a reply to Lynch *et al.*, *Journal of Epidemiology and Community Health*, 54: 411–13.

Wilkinson, R.G. (2005) Inequality: what it does and how to reduce it, in: *UK Health Watch 2005: The Experience of Health in an Unequal Society*. Politics of Health Group.

Woolcock, M. (2001) The place of social capital in understanding social and economic outcomes, *Canadian Journal of Policy Research*, 2(1).

15 Workplaces as settings for public health development

Paul Fleming

Work is recognized as one of the key social determinants of health (Marmot *et al.* 1999; Wilkinson and Marmot 2003; WHO 2005a). Its importance is located in the fact that it provides income that determines, to a great extent, the socioeconomic status of individuals, which in turn can have an effect on their health (Adler and Ostrove 1999; DoH 2004). Work also provides independence from support systems such as family and social welfare and determines the range of life chances available to individuals. Further, if levels of self direction permitted in the workplace are low, this can negatively affect attitudes and behaviour; these effects can extend into areas such as family and social life (Siegrist 2002).

Recent decades have seen some of the most radical changes in the nature of work and its organization (Landbergis 2003). This has been in no small measure due to the effects of globalization (see Chapter 10 for a full discussion of globalization). In the last quarter century, global economic and social influences have had a profound effect on the world of work with implications for the health of workers (Chu and Dwyer 2002). The economies of developed industrial nations in western Europe and North America have seen a steady shift from their traditional workplace strengths of heavy engineering and manufacturing to an IT and services oriented base. This has produced changes in social and economic structures that have led to decreases in job security, with an increasing proportion of the workforce being employed on a fixed term basis (Siegrist 2002). This has resulted in increasingly negative effects on the health of employees (Missler and Theuringer 2003). A shift has occurred in major workplace health issues as industrial accidents and conditions derived from exposure to pollutants decline and stress-related illness and the effects of ageing increase (Chu 2003). Those societies which have seen more recent development of their economic base, notably those in South and East Asia, have witnessed a rapid transition from subsistence farming to burgeoning industrial manufacturing and, increasingly, an IT-based economy. This changing environment of work is presenting major challenges for workplace health (see Chapter 5 for a more detailed examination of workplace health).

Since a large number of people spend a great deal of time at work, the workplace must be considered a key setting for public health action. This chapter explores how the settings approach to workplace health is a vehicle for empowerment of workforces and individual workers to achieve enhanced health status, identifying the benefits and issues for employers. The capacity of national workplace health promotion strategies to contribute to the reduction of inequalities in health will be examined and several examples of good practice considered.

The workplace as a setting for promoting health

The World Health Organization (WHO) has identified in target 13 of its *Health 21* strategy the need for settings for health (WHO 1999). More recently, the WHO has declared that the 'workplace, along with the school, hospital, city, island and marketplace, has been established as one of the priority settings for health promotion into the 21st Century' (WHO 2006: 1). The influence of the workplace on the physical, mental, economic and social wellbeing of workers is of considerable importance for population health. Benefits are identified for the employee which include 'a safe and healthy working environment, enhanced self esteem, reduced stress, improved morale, increased job satisfaction, increased skills for health protection, improved health and an improved sense of wellbeing' (WHO 2006: 2).

From the employer perspective, the WHO outlines benefits of the health promoting workplace for the employer to include 'a well managed health and safety programme, a positive and caring image, improved staff morale, turnover and absenteeism, increased productivity, and reduced health care/insurance costs and risk of fines and litigation' (WHO 2006: 2). The Faculties of Public Health (FPH) and Occupational Health (FOH) mirror these benefits to the UK in their employer focused publication *Creating a Healthy Workplace* (FPH/FOH 2006). It is significant that in many workplace health promotion initiatives, a recurrent theme is the selling of the concept of workplace health promotion to employers in the first instance. This appears to be in recognition of the fact that power is balanced in favour of the employer to decide whether or not to engage in a health-promoting workplace initiative (Health Canada 2001).

In the European context, the work of the European Network of Health Promoting Workplaces (ENHPW), which is funded by the European Union (EU), is central to an understanding of current workplace health promotion practice. In its Luxembourg Declaration, the ENHPW conceived workplace health as combining the efforts of employers, employees and society to improve the health and wellbeing of people at work through a combination of: improving work organization and the working environment; promoting active participation; and encouraging personal development (ENHPW 1997). This perspective was given further substance by the *Barcelona Declaration on Developing Good Workplace Practice in Europe* (ENHPW 2002). This declaration highlighted workplace health promotion as one of the drivers for social and economic success in Europe and encouraged the development of supportive infrastructure for the implementation of good workplace health promotion.

How is the goal of healthy employees in a healthy organization achieved through a settings approach? Broadly, a setting is any defined entity, organization or geographical area where a whole system approach can be adopted to the improvement of health at both the individual and population level. In most situations where a health-promoting workplace is being developed, it is assumed that the employer's responsibility is to develop policies that will provide an environment (physical, social and organizational) supportive to health. It is also, however, employees' responsibility to engage with their own wellbeing (Shain and Suurvali 2001).

The workplace, with its structural power imbalances between employers and employees (Spector 1998; Health Canada 2001), can make facilitating real partnership somewhat difficult. The increase of control necessary for health improvement, which is basic to health promotion (WHO 1986, 1997), may have implications for the empowerment agenda of people at work with regard to health improvement (Peltomäki *et al.* 2003; Arneson and Ekberg 2005). In terms of a social model of public health, empowerment can be facilitated through the principles of community defined health agendas. Building social capital, shared authority between providers and users of services and working in partnership with population groups are key strategies in this bottom-up approach (Dalziel 2003). Such principles underlie the Health and Safety Executive (HSE) for Great Britain's strategy for worker involvement in health and safety management (HSE 2004).

Building a health-promoting workplace through an empowered workforce and employer commitment provides particular challenges for the ethos of health promotion programme design. A number of models have been designed to facilitate understanding of the structure and interrelationships within the various elements of the health promoting workplace (for example Harvey and Fleming 2004; The Health Communications Unit 2004). See Figure 15.1 for a synthesis of a number of these. It is important to note that the key elements of the model are set in the context of a complex web of health determinants which include individual, job, organizational and external factors (LaBonte 1995). The latter factors provide the external operating environment, the environment of public policy (healthy and otherwise), societal and employment sector norms and, as indicated earlier, factors such as globalization.

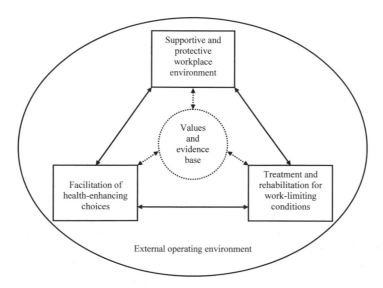

Figure 15.1   The health-promoting workplace

Values and evidence base

The notion of an appropriate values and evidence base, with the consequent ability to develop a coherent evaluation strategy, is central to the creation of the health-promoting workplace. It is particularly important that those who support capacity building in workplace health have a clear concept of an appropriate values base and are conversant with the evidence base that can be used to inform the development of health-promoting workplaces.

In terms of values (Guttmann 2000), a health-promoting workplace must be inclusive and facilitative in its approach and therefore equity, empowerment, respect and informed participation are foundational to the ethical development of the setting. An inclusive agenda will display a commitment to equity by facilitating empowerment through partnership between employer and employee in decision making in the workplace. Such an approach can contribute to the redressing of the effects of power imbalances between employer and employee, such as those which can be observed in workplaces where policy and practice can be changed without adequate consultation (St Leger 1997).

In addition to values, the complexity of needs assessment that contributes to an effective evidence base for the workplace setting remains a challenge (Fleming 1999). If the evidence base is to be inclusive, the concept of assessment of need for health promotion must take into account organizational, social and environmental concerns and address the issue of wellbeing (Tones and Green 2004). In a social model of public health it is essential to move beyond the disease focused approach to health assessment normally linked with the traditional epidemiological paradigm for needs assessment. Qualitative data that describe the experiences and perspectives of both employees and employers are a vital element of the evidence base. This is particularly so in a context where a setting such as the workplace needs to develop comprehensive, whole system approaches to be effective (Breuker and Schröer 2000). Planners can therefore monitor disease indicators of inequality, where conditions such as cardiovascular disease impact adversely on the workforce, particularly those who are socioeconomically disadvantaged. However, an equal emphasis can also be placed on the expressed health and wellbeing needs of the workforce and their preferred solutions (Robinson and Elkan 1996). The needs of people, in this case workers, are the primary guide for the equitable distribution of opportunities for health improvement (Nutbeam 1998). Hearing the voices of the workforce is fundamental to empowerment for health.

A further consideration in the development of an evidence base is the assembling of knowledge relating to the effectiveness of a range of approaches to promoting health in the workplace. At present, evaluation of settings is at a relatively early stage of development with defensible evaluation and research studies still being relatively rare (St Leger 1997). Further, the nature of the evidence base for health promotion practice is a matter of some debate. If evidence is understood to be facts and/or data which are employed in problem solving and decision making (McQueen and Anderson 2001) then the evidence base for the health-promoting workplace must be relatively eclectic. Further, evaluative evidence should be multi layered and focus on how the development of the whole system of the health-promoting workplace has contributed to health improvement. Addressing this level of complexity will avoid the possibility of adopting a reductionist approach to assembling an evidence base (Nutbeam 1999). However, at present the majority of eva- luative studies still tend to focus on individual initiatives undertaken within the context of the setting (Dugdill and Springett 2001), thus losing the added value of assessing the whole setting (Dooris 2006). If, however, evidence relating to the effects of specific in- terventions is gathered for its value in contributing to empowerment in the workplace, this would prove invaluable in planning for the health-promoting workplace (Arneson and Ekberg 2005).

Supportive and protective workplace environments

In moving to the three central, interlinked activity areas of the health-promoting workplace, the development of a supportive and protective workplace environment is fundamental to the setting. The concept of a supportive environment (WHO 1991) im- plies that the organizational and social environment in the workplace creates a workplace culture that facilitates health development in the workforce. Thus organizational issues such as flexible working, organization of work practices, development of opportunities for personal development and the creation and maintenance of a pleasant physical en- vironment all contribute to a supportive environment. Partnership approaches between workforce and management will take these measures forward in an empowering manner that benefits all.

In terms of a protective environment, health and safety is the domain which is perhaps most closely associated with workplace health protection and has its roots in legislation and enforcement activity. The pervasiveness of health and safety in the workplace in contributing to a supportive workplace environment (Wright 1998) can be simply explained because it is a statutory imperative (Harvey and Fleming 2004). This element of the health-promoting workplace seeks to prevent work related accidents and illness, thus reducing sickness absence rates in a number of key conditions with con- sequent positive effects on productivity. These conditions include musculo-skeletal disorders, stress related illness, respiratory and skin conditions (Harvey and Fleming 2004). There has been some anxiety that, in some instances, health and safety has re- ceived undue emphasis to the exclusion of wider health promotion initiatives. However, given that health and safety has had a longer time to embed in the culture of the workplace, it is hardly surprising that the much newer concept of the health-promoting workplace is taking time to become established across all employment sectors, both in large employers and with small and medium-sized enterprises (SMEs).

Treatment and rehabilitation

Treatment and rehabilitation involves assisting those with a specific illness or disability to engage or re-engage with work in a manner appropriate to their health status (Disler and Palant 2001; British Society of Rehabilitation Medicine 2003). The key aim here is to recognize that most people wish to work, even those who have not worked for some time (Secker and Membrey 2003). Waiting until a condition is completely resolved may not always result in the most positive outcome in terms of returning to work and thus economic productivity (WHO 1994; DoH 2004). While it is to the benefit of the employee to be at full potential at the earliest possible opportunity, this element of the health-promoting workplace tends to have a strong driver from the employer perspective to maintain maximum productivity levels through the reduction of sickness absence levels. People are either treated in order to prevent absence occurring or are rehabilitated to ensure their return to work at the earliest possible opportunity. It was in this context, therefore, that in 1994, the Beijing Declaration stated the right of all workers to have access to occupational health services (WHO 1994). It is also an interesting example of the interface between a social determinant of health, in this case work, and a more biomedical approach to addressing health deficits.

Facilitation of health-enhancing choices in the workplace

Facilitation of health-enhancing choices is the element of the health-promoting workplace that is perhaps most closely linked in the public mind with health promotion. This perception often focuses on high-profile elements of lifestyle issues, sometimes described as health practices (Health Canada 1998), such as healthy eating and physical activity. However, if healthy choices are to be made, those engaged in the choosing often need to be empowered to make appropriate choices (Koelen and Lindstrom 2005). We need to recognize that healthier choices go beyond lifestyle into issues such as choosing flexible work patterns which best fit with other areas of life, such as responsibilities as carers. Wage and salary levels also contribute to health choices in that they influence other health determinants such as housing, transport and access to leisure facilities. The impact of the workplace is therefore far reaching in terms of health related choice.

To understand how the health-promoting workplace concept operates, a number of key questions should be asked when assessing any health-promoting workplace at the organizational/business level. First, is a whole systems approach adopted which is based on considered values and an evidence base and where all strategic elements receive balanced attention? Are the employees in health promoting workplaces sufficiently empowered individually and collectively in their working lives to enhance their health status both inside and outside work? Are genuine partnership approaches in use, where the voices of employer and employee can be equally heard? Does the time and effort expended by the employer justify the investment in terms of positive returns for the organization/business? Finally, are the process, impact and outcome of health-promoting approaches appropriately evaluated to ascertain their efficiency and effectiveness?

Key initiatives in health-promoting workplaces

The concept of the health-promoting workplace has generated a range of responses both nationally and internationally. The ENHPW has developed within its Healthy Employees in Healthy Organizations initiative the ENHPW Toolbox, a collection of methods and practices for promoting health at the workplace (ENHPW 2004). This approach has seen the development of a wide range of tools that can be programmes, projects (models of good practice) or instruments (questionnaires, guidelines and information materials). These tools can be applied in a wide range of contexts in terms of employer size and type of employment sector. They are also applied to a range of health policy issues in the workplace, such as work–life balance or gender equality and/or lifestyle issues such as smoking and nutrition. In terms of good health promotion practice, this initiative has developed a set of quality standards that enable formal evaluations to be undertaken both in larger organizations (ENHPW 1999) and in SMEs (ENHPW 2001a, 2001b). The Toolbox draws on a range of initiatives from 22 countries but, while many of these have undergone early development and dissemination, there appears to be a paucity of formal independent evaluation in a number of the projects and tools published. Further, the level of reporting makes it difficult to understand how well, in some cases, the projects are embedded in a whole systems approach in the workplaces in which they have been implemented.

In the wider international context, the federal government of Canada is perhaps one of the best known and well established in this field. In Canada, workplace health has been addressed by approaches tailored to the workplace sector. Three models based on a whole systems approach have been developed, namely the corporate health model, the small business health model and the farm health model (Health Canada 1996). While the corporate model focuses on establishing the concept of a health-promoting workplace in a single organization, the small business and farm models depend on the development and facilitation of coalitions of interested parties, both employer and employee, by local health promotion agencies. These latter models use groups of SMEs or farm operators to develop critical mass for effective provision of support for workplace health promotion. All three models emphasize employee participation and partnerships between interested parties who would wish to develop the health-promoting workplace. When the health-promoting workplace concept is established, each of the three models advocates common elements such as: needs assessment; the development of workplace health profiles; business health plans appropriate to the sector (two to three years for SMEs and farms and three to five years for the corporate sector); programme action plans (annual); and progress reviews.

Health Canada has, in addition to disseminating the health models, commissioned research that has identified factors that contribute positively to the health of employees. These include organizational issues such as leadership which values employees, employee participation, job control, communication, learning opportunities, commitment to work–life balance and individual wellness (Lowe 2003). This study also suggests that there are positive, causal links between the creation of healthy workplaces, the health status of employees and productivity at the company level. Further, healthy workplace initiatives are perceived to be comprehensive, integrated into human resource programmes with implementation strategies that are characterized by strong leadership, good communication and widespread participation. Overall, this research affirms the principles on which health-promoting workplaces are based.

In the UK, workplace health promotion has been established as a key target for public health interventions through several White Papers on public health. In England, *Choosing Health: Making Healthy Choices Easier* (DoH 2004) is the current driver for workplace health promotion, a complete chapter of the White Paper being devoted to the issue of work and health. Similar approaches have been adopted in Scotland (Scottish Executive 2003) and in Northern Ireland (DHSSPS 2002).

In *Choosing Health: Making Healthy Choices Easier*, employment is seen as key to improving health and reducing inequalities. The interplay between personal choices made by people at work and the effects that the work environment and organization has on these choices is recognized. The desire of the government to reduce health and disability benefit levels, derived from its welfare reform agenda, also pervades the document. As is often the case with government strategy documents, the positive outcomes of national employment and health policies are presented in a somewhat uncritical manner. For instance, lone parents gaining paid employment through the New Deal initiative, the first phase of welfare reform in the UK, is presented as a positive outcome of government policy. However, there is little recognition of the balance between the positive outcomes, such as increased income and non-dependence on benefits, and negative outcomes, such as stresses involved in accessing suitable, affordable childcare and achieving appropriate work–life balance. Inequalities may be addressed through improvement in income but does the increase in earnings, even when supplemented by a range of benefits, bring a justifiable net gain to the quality of life?

In a parallel development, *Health, Work and Wellbeing* has been jointly developed by the Department of Work and Pensions (DWP) and the Department of Health (DoH) and the HSE (DWP 2005). Given the composition of this collaboration, it is no surprise that this strategy also has a major focus on improving working lives through healthy workplaces as a contribution to the welfare reform agenda. The agenda is underpinned by three stated ways in which individuals can benefit from the strategy. These are to help people manage minor health problems at work, avoid work related health problems and return to health following an absence from work because of illness. While these three elements are, in themselves, laudable for employees, it is also obvious that the primary focus has major benefits for both employers, by reducing absence and increasing productivity, and for government, by reducing claims on the benefits system and pressures on the health and social services. This approach is indicative of an ethos that creates a tension between the concepts of empowerment and participation for workers and the wider context of government social and economic policy driven by economic expediency.

The current movement for health improvement in the workplace goes back, however, to earlier public health initiatives, notably *Saving Lives: Our Healthier Nation* (DoH 1999). This White Paper confirmed the trend towards joined up thinking for the development of workplace health policy. The HSE, which is responsible along with local authorities for enforcement of health and safety legislation in Great Britain, has had a central role in this process. It has provided the unifying thread for the development of the Healthy Workplace Initiative (HSE 1999), a workplace health promotion strategy in partnership with health departments in England, Scotland and Wales.

The Healthy Workplace Initiative

The Healthy Workplace Initiative was designed to improve health and reduce inequalities in health. The underlying principle of the initiative was to establish health as an integral element of businesses' thinking and organizational development, a whole systems approach. Since 2000, the Healthy Workplace Initiative has been at the forefront of an array of strategies, including the development of NHS Plus, a project providing access to NHS occupational health services for non NHS SMEs, and *Securing Health Together*, an occupational health strategy which stops workers becoming ill and facilitates those who do become ill to re-enter the workforce as quickly as possible.

Improvement of the health and safety element of workplace health has also been a high priority with the *Revitalizing Health and Safety Strategy* and the *Strategy for Health and Safety in Great Britain to 2010 and Beyond* (HSE 2004), the latter being built on Securing Health Together. Other strategies outside the Healthy Workplace Initiative include the Department of Trade and Industry's (DTI) Work–life Balance Campaign (DTI 2003, 2004) and the Home Office's Business Engagement Strategy (Home Office 2002) which contains an element of addressing drug use in the workplace. This extensive range of initiatives, along with parallel strategies in Scotland and Wales and, in addition, many workplace health promotion initiatives at regional and local levels, might be a sign of too many initiatives being delivered within too short a time span.

Developing the health-promoting workplace

This plethora of strategies has produced a significant level of activity in the workplace health promotion field, but have they worked? Strategies deriving from the Healthy Workplace Initiative use approaches which reflect the WHO assertion that awards for the development of health-promoting workplaces can be helpful (WHO 2005b). Scotland has developed the Healthy Working Lives programme (Scottish Executive 2004), which now contains within it the well-established Scotland's Health at Work (SHAW 2006) award for employers who wish to be recognized for their efforts in workplace health promotion. This award can be gained at bronze, silver and gold levels, each level displaying increasing sophistication in the level of engagement with workplace health promotion. Like the Canadian models, the SHAW initiative provides local advisers to assist employers with the development of workplace health promotion strategies.

A similar initiative has been developed in Wales through the Health at Work initiative with its Corporate Health Standard award, which, like the Scottish award, is offered at several levels (National Assembly for Wales 2005). Here the bronze standard of award is given for evidence of work in the core components of policy development, organizational support, employee involvement and communication. In addition, the employer must have in place measures relating to health and safety, tobacco use, musculo-skeletal disorders, mental health and alcohol and substance misuse; either nutrition or physical activity will also be chosen at this level. Thereafter, the silver, gold and platinum awards acknowledge increasing complexity and challenge in each of these areas, with the latter focusing particularly on the area of corporate social responsibility. The advantage of this type of award is that, while specific health topics may receive precedence at specific points in time, an underlying whole system approach is necessary for the award to be achieved. A more cynical view might suggest that the reputational advantage gained by such awards may not always be reflected in the reality of day-to-day organizational behaviour.

In Northern Ireland, which sits outside the workplace health structures of Great Britain, developments regarding workplace health promotion are interesting as this is a region with a small population. The province has a relatively weak economy with a high percentage of SMEs as employers (about 99 per cent) and a higher than average dependence for employment on the public sector. As in Great Britain, a key partnership for workplace health promotion is found at the regional level between the Health Promotion Agency for Northern Ireland and the Health and Safety Executive for Northern Ireland (HSENI). They have developed the Working for Health strategy (HSENI 2003). This strategy has inspired the Work Well initiative for SMEs. A recent pilot study evaluation has shown that SMEs can facilitate improvements in personal health choices, the working environment and health and safety at work (HPANI 2006). Employers cited lack of time and competing priorities to be the greatest barriers to the development of health-promoting workplaces.

The ENHPW has also recognized good practice in a number of examples of health promoting workplace initiatives which have taken place in the UK context (ENHPW 2006). One of these was the Northern Ireland Court Service, a public-sector employer with fewer than 1000 employees. A workplace health promotion project was developed through its Workplace Health Unit by establishing a workplace health committee. This committee, which had strong backing from the organization's management board, was instrumental in establishing cooperation and communication structures and disseminating a tool, Discovering the Needs, based on the Canadian workplace health model. The findings resulted in a corporate action plan which focused on improving health through addressing stress in the social environment, health and safety management and a range of health topics which included nutrition, smoking, medication use, drinking and health practices. Workplace health assessments were accessed by 71 per cent of staff and a study of 50 of these staff members showed that significant changes had been made to diet and increases in the duration and frequency of physical activity. Relax and De-stress Workshops were well attended, and work on mental wellbeing and short-term absenteeism was ongoing at the time of reporting. Overall, this is a good example of a whole system approach where the organization paid attention to developing supportive and protective work environments, facilitated healthy personal choices and provided health assessment with remediation where appropriate. Commitment from the organization and senior management was a key element of the strategy.

This is but one of a plethora of examples of good practice which are publicized by the various organizations which aim to promote health in the workplace. The overall literature on evaluation of the health-promoting workplace is, however, weak. Many of the studies published focus on single issues such as back pain or nutrition and do not always comment on the contribution to addressing inequalities; many are not peer reviewed. In order to advance the state of knowledge that underpins good practice in implementing health-promoting workplace strategies, there is a need for well funded, defensible evaluation strategies. These strategies need to give a balanced picture of the effects the settings approach has on both employees and employers in order to encourage outcomes of enhancing empowerment and reducing inequalities in the workforce. They should also contribute to productivity in the workplace and economic growth at all levels of society. There is great potential in further developing the health-promoting workplace concept as an integral element of good public health practice in a rapidly changing world.

References

Adler, N.E. and Ostrove, J.M. (1999) Socioeconomic status and health: what we know and what we don't, *Annals of the New York Academy of Sciences*, 869: 3.

Arneson, H. and Ekberg, K. (2005) Evaluation of empowerment processes in a workplace health promotion intervention based on learning in Sweden, *Health Promotion International*, 20(4): 351–9.

Breuker, G. and Schröer, A. (2000) Settings 1 – health promotion in the workplace, in *Effective Health Promotion in the Workplace: The Evidence of Health Promotion Effectiveness, Shaping Public Health in a new Europe*. Vanves, France: International Union for Health Promotion and Education.

British Society of Rehabilitation Medicine (2003) *Vocational Rehabilitation – The Way Forward: Report of a Working Party*, 2nd edn. London: British Society of Rehabilitation Medicine.

Chu, C. (2003) *From Workplace Health Promotion to Integrative Workplace Health Management: Trends and Developments*. Geneva: GOHNET newsletter.

Chu, C. and Dwyer, S. (2002) Employer role in integrative workplace health management: a new model in progress, *Disease Management and Health Outcomes*, 10(3): 175–86.

Dalziel, Y. (2003) The role of nurses in public health, in A. Watterson (ed.) *Public Health Practice*. Basingstoke: Palgrave Macmillan.

DHSSPS (Department of Health, Social Services and Public Safety) (Northern Ireland) (2002) *Investing for Health*. Belfast: DHSSPS.

Disler, P.B. and Pallant, J.F. (2001) Vocational rehabilitation – everybody gains if injured workers are helped back into work, *British Medical Journal*, 323(7305): 121–3.

Dooris, M. (2006) Healthy settings: challenges to generating evidence of effectiveness, *Health Promotion International*, 21(1): 55–65.

DoH (Department of Health) (1999) *Saving Lives: Our Healthier Nation*. London: The Stationery Office.

DoH (Department of Health) (2004) *Choosing Health: Making Healthy Choices Easier*. London: The Stationery Office.

DTI (Department of Trade and Industry) (2003) *The Second Work–life Balance Study: Results from the Employees' Survey*, www.dti.gov.uk/files/file11513.pdf?pubpdfdload=03%2F1252, accessed 28 April 2006.

DTI (Department of Trade and Industry) (2004) *The Second Work–life Balance Study: Results from the Employees' Survey* www.dti.gov.uk/files/file11499.pdf?pubpdfdload=04%2F740, accessed 28 April 2006.

Dugdill, L. and Springett, J. (2001) Evaluating health promotion programmes in the workplace, in I. Rootman *et al.* (eds) *Evaluation in Health Promotion: Principles and Perspectives*. Copenhagen: WHO Regional Office for Europe.

DWP (Department of Work and Pensions) (2005) *Health, Work and wellbeing – Caring for Our Future*, www.dwp.gov.uk/publications/dwp/2005/health_and_wellbeing.pdf, accessed 28 April 2006.

ENHPW (European Network of Health Promoting Workplaces) (1997) *Luxembourg Declaration on Workplace Health Promotion in the European Union*. Luxembourg: European Network of Health Promoting Workplaces.

ENHPW (European Network of Health Promoting Workplaces) (1999) *Quality Criteria of Workplace Health Promotion*. Essen: European Network of Health Promoting Workplaces.

ENHPW (European Network of Health Promoting Workplaces) (2001a) *The Lisbon Statement on Workplace Health in SMEs*. Lisbon: European Network of Health Promoting Workplaces.

ENHPW (European Network of Health Promoting Workplaces) (2001b) *Small, Healthy and Competitive – New Strategies for Improved Health in SMEs*. Essen: European Network of Health Promoting Workplaces.

ENHPW (European Network of Health Promoting Workplaces) (2002) *The Barcelona Declaration on Developing Good Workplace Health Practice in Europe*. Barcelona: European Network of Health Promoting Workplaces.

ENHPW (European Network of Health Promoting Workplaces) (2004) *ENHPW Toolbox*, www.enwhp.org/whp/whp-models-good-practice-country.php.

ENHPW (European Network of Health Promoting Workplaces) (2006) *Models of Good Practice by Country* www.enwhp.org/whp/whp-models-good-practice-country.php.

Fleming, P. (1999) Health promotion for individuals, families and communities, in A. Long (ed.) *Interactions for Practice in Community Nursing*. Basingstoke: Macmillan.

FPH/FOH (Faculty of Public Health/Faculty of Occupational Health) (2006) *Creating a Healthy Workplace*. London: Faculty of Public Health/Faculty of Occupational Health.

Guttmann, N. (2000) *Public Health Communication Interventions: Values and Ethical Dilemmas*. Thousand Oaks, CA: Sage.

Harvey, H. and Fleming, P. (2004) *Impacting Health at Work*. London: Chadwick House Publishing.

Health Canada (1996) *Workplace Health Strategies*, www.hc-sc.gc.ca/ewh-semt/occup-travail/work-travail/wh-mat-strategies_e.html, accessed 28 April 2006.

Health Canada (1998) *Workplace Health System – Influencing Employee Health*. Ottawa: Health Canada.

Health Canada (2001) *Fairness in Families, Schools and Workplaces: Implications for Healthy Relationships in these Environments*. Ottawa: Health Canada.

Health Communications Unit, the (2004) *Influencing the Organisational Environment to Create Healthy Workplaces*. Toronto: The Health Communication Unit.

Home Office (2002) *Drug Strategy – Drugs in the Workplace*, www.drugs.gov.uk/drug-strategy/drugs-in-workplace, accessed: 28 April 2006.

HPANI (Health Promotion Agency for Northern Ireland) (2006) *Summary Evaluation of the Work Well Initiative*. Belfast: HPANI.

HSE Health and Safety Executive (1999) *About the Healthy Workplace Initiative*, www.signup web.net, accessed 28 April 2006.

HSE Health and Safety Executive (2004) *Worker Involvement in Health and Safety Management*. London: HSE.

HSENI (Health and Safety Executive for Northern Ireland) (2003) *Working for Health*. Belfast: HSENI.

Koelen, M.A. and Lindstrom, B. (2005) Making healthy choices easy choices: the role of empowerment, *European Journal of Clinical Nutrition*, 59 Suppl: S10–5, discussion S16, S23.

Labonte, R. (1995) Population health and health promotion: what do they have to say to each other? *Canadian Journal of Public Health*, 86(3): 165–8.

Landsbergis, P.A. (2003) The changing organisation of work and the safety and health of working people: a commentary, *Journal of Occupational & Environmental Medicine*, 45(1): 61–72.

Lowe, G.S. (2003) *Healthy Workplaces and Productivity: A Discussion Paper*. Ottawa: Economic Analysis and Evaluation Division, Health Canada.

Marmot, M., Siegrist, J., Theorell, T. and Feeney, A. (1999) Health and the psychosocial environment at work, in M.G. Marmot and R.G. Wilkinson (eds) *The Social Determinants of Health*. Oxford: Oxford University Press.

McQueen, D. and Anderson, L. (2001) What counts as evidence: issues and debates, in I. Rootman *et al.* (eds) *Evaluation in Health Promotion: Principles and Perspectives*. Copenhagen: WHO Regional Office for Europe.

Missler, M. and Theuringer, T. (2003) Brave new working world? Europe needs investment in workplace health promotion more than ever before, Promotion and Education, X(4): 5.

National Assembly for Wales (2005) *Corporate Health Standard*. Cardiff: Health and Social Care.

Nutbeam, D. (1998) Evaluating health promotion – progress, problems and solutions, *Health Promotion International*, 13(1): 27–43.

Nutbeam, D. (1999) The challenge to provide 'evidence' in health promotion, *Health Promotion International*, 14(2): 99–101.

Peltomäki, P., Johansson, M., Ahrens, W., Sala, M., Wesseling, F.B. and Berenes, F. (2003) Social context for workplace health promotion: feasibility considerations in Costa Rica, Finland, Germany, Spain and Sweden, *Health Promotion International*, 18(2): 115–26.

Robinson, J. and Elkan, R. (1996) *Health Needs Assessment: Theory and Practice*. London: Churchill Livingstone.

Scottish Executive (2003) *Improving Health in Scotland – The Challenge*. Edinburgh: Scottish Executive.

Scottish Executive (2004) *Healthy Working Lives*. Edinburgh: Scottish Executive.

Shain, M. and Suurvali, H. (2001) *Investing in Comprehensive Workplace Health Promotion*. Toronto: National Quality Institute.

SHAW (Scotland's Health at Work) (2006) www.shaw.uk.com, accessed 28 April 2006.

Siegrist, J. (2002) Reducing social inequalities in health: work-related strategies, *Scandinavian Journal of Public Health*, 30(Supp. 59): 49–53.

Spector, P.E. (1998) A control theory of the job stress process, in C.E. Cooper (ed.) *Theories of Organisational Stress*. Oxford: Oxford University Press.

St Leger, L. (1997) Health promoting settings: from Ottawa for Jakarta, *Health Promotion International*, 12(2): 99–100.

Tones, K. and Green, J. (2004) *Health Promotion Planning and Settings*. London: Sage.

WHO (World Health Organization) (1986) *Ottawa Charter for Health Promotion*. Geneva: World Health Organization.

WHO (World Health Organization) (1991) *Sundsvall Statement on Supportive Environments for Health*. Copenhagen: World Health Organization Regional Office for Europe.

WHO (World Health Organization) (1994) *Declaration on Occupational Health for All*. Beijing: World Health Organization.

WHO (World Health Organization) (1997) *Jakarta Declaration on Health Promotion*. Jakarta: World Health Organization.

WHO (World Health Organization) (1999) *Health 21: Health for All in the 21st Century*. Copenhagen: World Health Organization Regional Office for Europe.

WHO (World Health Organization) (2005a) *The Bangkok Charter for Health Promotion in a Globalised World*. Geneva: World Health Organization.

WHO (World Health Organization) (2005b) *Action on the Social Determinants of Health – Learning from Previous Experiences*. Geneva: World Health Organization.

WHO (World Health Organization) (2006) *Workplace Health Promotion*. Geneva: World Health Organization.

Wilkinson, R. and Marmot, M. (eds) (2003) *The Solid Facts*. Copenhagen: World Health Organization.

Wright, M.S. (1998) *Factors Motivating Proactive Health and Safety Management*. HSE CRR1998:179. Sudbury: HSE Books.

16 Healthy Cities: key principles for professional practice

Roderick Lawrence and Colin Fudge

In 1987, the World Health Organization (WHO) Regional Office for Europe in conjunction with 11 cities founded the Healthy Cities project. Today there are more than 30 national and regional networks in Europe involving about 600 municipalities, complemented by many hundreds more in each of the regions of the world (see www.euro.who.int/healthy-cities).

The central purpose of this chapter is to consider the basis of the Healthy Cities programme. The fundamental principles and strategies on which the programme is based will be examined and conclusions drawn about the effectiveness and the future of the Healthy Cities initiative as public health action.

What is a healthy city?

The Healthy Cities programme is based on the principles and strategies of Health for All (HFA) (see http://www.euro.who.int/AboutWHO/Policy/20010827_1 and WHO 1998), which emphasizes prevention of diseases, intersectoral cooperation and community participation. The Ottawa Charter (WHO 1986) provides the strategic framework for HFA and therefore directly influences the Healthy Cities movement through the Ottawa principles of healthy public policies, creating supportive environments, strengthening community participation, improving personal skills and reorientating health services (see Chapter 11 for further discussion of healthy public policies). Agenda 21 (UN 1992), the global programme of action on sustainable development, is also central to Healthy Cities. The fundamental goal of the Healthy Cities programme is to provide an effective means of dealing with health-related aspects of poverty, pollution, lifestyle changes, urban planning, transport and the special needs of marginalized and vulnerable groups in urban areas (see for an example of this, www.afro.who.int/eph/publications/brochure_reducing-poverty-hcp.pdf). Strategies used within Healthy Cities include integrating health into multiple-sector policy agendas, creating strong partnerships for health between groups in the public and private sectors, and the use of participatory approaches (Werna *et al.* 1998, 1999; WHO 2000c).

The Healthy Cities programme in the WHO European region includes four main components:

1   designated cities that are committed to a comprehensive approach to achieving the goals of the programme;

2   national and sub national networks that facilitate, together with EURONET, cooperation between partners;

3   multi city action plans (MCAPs) implemented by networks of cities collaborating on specific issues of common interest;

4   model projects in central and eastern Europe.

Supported by WHO collaborating centres and operating alongside the European Sustainable City policy agenda (http://ec.europa.eu/environment/urban/locsm-en.htm), the Healthy Cities initiative is mainly concerned with the interrelations between living conditions and the health of the residents in urban areas (Green *et al.* 2003). While there are close links and common agendas between Healthy Cities and European Sustainable Cities, collaboration has not been optimized as it might have been (Fudge 2004).

Principles of the WHO Healthy Cities programme

Table 16.1   Principles that underpin a healthy city

1 Meeting basic needs (for food, water shelter, income, safety and work) for all the city's people
2 A clean, safe physical environment of high quality, including housing quality
3 An ecosystem that is stable now and sustainable in the long term
4 A diverse, vital and innovative economy
5 A mutually supportive and non exploitive community
6 A high degree of participation and control by the public over the decisions affecting their lives, health and wellbeing
7 The encouragement of connectedness with the past, with the cultural and biological heritage of city dwellers and with other groups and individuals
8 Access to a wide variety of experiences and resources with the chance for a wide variety of contact, interaction and communications
9 A built form that is compatible with and enhances the preceding characteristics
10 An optimum level of appropriate public health and sick care services accessible to all
11 High health status (high levels of positive health and low levels of disease)

Source: diverse WHO publications and Goldstein (2000)

The following 11 fundamental principles characterize healthy cities (see Table 16.1 for a summary).

1   *The meeting of basic needs* is paramount, including the supply of fundamental resources, food, water, shelter, income, safety and work, and the secure disposal of all kinds of solid and liquid wastes. This is a challenging principle as, to take one example, the large majority of urban populations in the world are totally dependent on imported foods from far beyond the hinterland of their city. In 2000, only an estimated 15 to 20 per cent of all food in the world was produced in urban areas. The WHO estimates that around 30 per cent of the world population suffers from one or more of the numerous kinds of malnutrition, and that urban populations are disproportionately at risk (WHO 2000b). An integrated approach to food production and consumption, environmental quality, sustainable resource use and health can be achieved by policies that promote the local production of fresh foods (Barton and Tsourou 2000; Fudge 2003a). Urban agriculture can help address nutrition deficiencies, reduce the risk of food borne and possibly other noncommunicable diseases, promote food security and ensure that urban populations have physical and economic access to enough food for an active, healthy life. Food security entails sustainable food production and consumption, governed by principles of equity, that the food is nutritionally adequate and personally and culturally acceptable, and that food is obtained and consumed in a matter that upholds basic human dignity (Pederson *et al.* 2000).

2   *A clean, safe physical environment of high quality* involves protection from natural disasters such as earthquakes, landslides, flooding and fires and from any potential source of natural radon (WHO 1997). The built environment should provide a shelter from the extremes of outdoor temperature; a protection against dust, insects and rodents; security from unwanted persons; insulation against noise and other pollutants and the local climate (Schwela 2000). Occupancy conditions in buildings, notably population density in residential buildings, is also a significant issue as it influences the transmission of airborne infections and the incidence of injury from domestic accidents (Gray 2001). The physical environment should also permit easy access to community facilities and services (for commerce, education, employment, leisure and primary healthcare) that are affordable and available to all individuals and groups irrespective of age, socio-economic status, ethnicity or religion (WHO 2000a). Other issues include the control of vectors and hosts of disease outdoors and inside buildings which can propagate in the building structure; the use of non toxic materials and finishes for building construction; the use and storage of hazardous substances or equipment in the urban environment (WHO 1990). In addition to the above, research in environmental psychology during the 1990s confirms that the relations between urban environments and health are not limited to the physical environment. Residential areas ought to be considered in terms of their capacity to nurture and sustain social and psychological processes (Gabe and Williams 1993; Halpern 1995; Ludermir and Harpham 1998; DETR 1999). The multiple dimensions of residential environments that circumscribe a resident's capacity to use their domestic setting to promote wellbeing is a subject that has been studied by a limited number of scholars during the last decade (Ekblad 1993; Halpern 1995). Studies in several industrialized countries show that more than

half of all non sleep activities of employed people between 18 and 64 years of age occur inside housing units. Certain groups, such as young children and the retired, spend even more time indoors. Consequently, their prolonged exposure to shortcomings in the indoor residential environment may have strong impacts on their health and wellbeing.

3   *An ecosystem that is stable now and sustainable in the long term* has direct implications for the construction of new cities or urban neighbourhoods, signifying the need for careful appraisal of the constituents of the local environment. Explicit land use guidelines and policies should avoid flood plains, seismic faults and dangers from landslides, while preserving wildlife habitat and agricultural fields in the hinterlands (Barton and Tsourou 2000; Fudge and Rowe 2000; Fudge 2005). Sites chosen for future urban development must incur the fewest ecological, economic and social costs. Consequently, new cities and urban neighbourhoods can be developed in a way that preserves the ecological infrastructure underlying the human settlement, especially genetic diversity, soil fertility, mineral reserves and water catchment areas. During the period 1990–9 more than 186 million people lost their homes due to natural or human-made disasters. What is also notable in these cases of natural disasters is that injury and death are disproportionately high among low-income groups who live on sloping sites prone to landslides, or in residential buildings least able to withstand tremors (UNCHS 1996; Mitchell 1999). During the twentieth century, issues related to economic and population growth, the accumulation and distribution of capital and material goods, as well as managing the interrelations between public and private interests dominated social development and urban policies in many countries. For example, Sweden is a recognized leader in its commitment to environmental protection, ecological technological innovation and high levels of healthcare and welfare provision. However, even in Sweden, a schism seems to be developing with key economic drivers. Policy agendas are increasingly difficult to join up and integrative policies between health and spatial planning are difficult to implement (Fudge and Rowe 2001). This means that the health and wellbeing of current and future generations, as well as the ecological impacts of urbanization, have not been a high priority.

4   *A diverse, vital and innovative economy.* Urbanization is a process that has been considered in relation to the economic growth of national economies and the global economy (Duffy 1995). In some countries, cities are locations for about two-thirds of gross domestic product (GDP). During the last three decades, those countries that urbanized most rapidly also had the highest levels of economic growth (UNCHS 1996). These trends have also led to relatively high levels of urban poverty and limited achievements in improving environmental conditions including a sufficient volume of potable water and effective site drainage, and sewage and solid waste disposal, with consequent negative impacts on health (Lee 1999). It is important to consider all feasible development options alongside their environmental, economic, health and other social impacts (Lawrence 1995). For example, economic incentives to promote local

employment by constructing new factories in a city may be successful in creating jobs, while simultaneously permitting emissions that have negative impacts on the quality of air and local water supplies in that locality and adjoining areas.

5   *A strong, mutually supportive and non-exploitive community* reflects equity, a key concept of the WHO Healthy Cities project (Goldstein 2000; Tsouros and Farrington 2003). Equity refers to justice and fair conduct and implies fairness in the relationship between individuals, population groups and the state. These relationships include a just distribution of the benefits and services in a society with respect to a universal standard or values such as human rights. For example, no individual or institution should act in a way to damage, compromise or limit the freedom and rights of others. Equity is an important component of the division of capital, as well as access to and distribution of information, resources and services including education, healthcare and social welfare (Lawrence 2002). The distinction between equality and equity is important because equality means equal circumstances, treatment and outcomes for all, whereas equity recognizes social differences and seeks to establish whether these differences are fair and just (see McDaid and Oliver 2005: 13 for further discussion of the implications of equality and equity). Inequalities of professional status, income, housing and work conditions are reflected in and reinforced by inequalities of health and wellbeing (WHO 2005). Although the economic, social and physical characteristics of urban neighbourhoods can be correlated with rates of morbidity and mortality, the lifestyle of groups and individuals cannot be ignored (Marmot and Wilkinson 1999). Residents in deprived urban areas commonly have poorer diets and smoking is also more prevalent, especially among women (Wilkinson 1996). In essence when poverty is interpreted as a compound index of deprivation including lack of income and lack of access to education, employment, housing and social support, it is a significant indicator of urban morbidity and mortality.

6   *A high degree of participation and control by the public over the decisions affecting their lives, health and wellbeing* is a prerequisite for a healthy city (WHO 2002). The term participation has a wide range of meanings because it can be interpreted as a means of achieving a goal or objective, and as a dynamic process that is not quantifiable or predictable. In the health sector, participation can be interpreted in a number of ways (see Scriven 2007 for a fuller discussion of community participation) and generally refers to dialogue between policy institutions and civic society about goals, projects and the allocation of resources to achieve desired outcomes. A wide range of techniques and methods can be used including civic forums, focus groups, citizens' juries, surveys, role playing and gaming (Barton and Tsourou 2000). Alongside the principle of participation an interest in the concept and practice of empowerment has developed in community development and urban planning. Empowerment is explicitly linked to citizen control in public and community health. Today, there is no shared definition of empowerment. Some argue that it is not normative because it is defined only in terms of its societal context. Nonetheless, the core of

empowerment includes the concepts of authority and power. These enable a process by which individuals and communities assume power and then act effectively in changing their lives and their local environment. Laverack (2004) points to the overlap between community empowerment and other concepts and processes such as community capacity building and community capital (see Chapters 6 and 14). The important point being made is that communities can gain power as a result of a change in control over the decisions that influence their lives. It is the communities themselves who achieve these outcomes by seizing or gaining power through a process of identifying problems and then implementing actions to solve them (Laverack 2001; Scriven 2007). Public participation and empowerment can serve as vehicles for identifying what local residents consider as key issues concerning the promotion of health and wellbeing. It is precisely this understanding that can lead to a reappraisal of separate policies from town planning and health that need to be more integrated (Barton and Tsourou 2000).

7   *The encouragement of connectedness with the past, with the cultural and biological heritage of city dwellers and with other groups and individuals* is commonly associated with the biological and ecological components of the urban location. The cultural heritage of cities is often considered in relation to human made monuments, public buildings and cultural festivals. However, in addition to these, urban history can be used creatively as a warehouse of knowledge, including the achievements and shortcomings of specific urban development projects, in order to build healthier cities. One positive lesson from urban history could be learnt from the public health reform movement that began in Britain in the nineteenth century following rapid urban population growth and industrialization. The public health problems of unsanitary housing, lack of a supply of safe water, ineffective sewage and solid waste disposal were related to health inequalities that were tackled by devolving responsibility and authority to local municipalities in Britain in 1866 (Fudge 2003b). The important role of local public administrations should be remembered at the beginning of the twenty first century when neoliberalism seems to have replaced state initiatives in many countries. It is appropriate to stress the need for public health interventions including solid waste disposal, sewage and water services, and affordable health service and medical care. In many countries today, including those in the former Soviet Union (see Godinho 2005), local public administrations lack the human and financial resources to counteract conditions in cities that have negative impacts on health and wellbeing.

8   *Access to a wide variety of experiences and resources with the chance for a wide variety of contact, interaction and communication* identifies the city as the focal point of creativity and culture; of conviviality and as a place for sedentary living. Cities of the twenty first century should not only be important hubs for national economic development but also functionally rich, having a sense of security and being people friendly. Social development is a key component of the WHO Healthy Cities project, which challenges quantified, economic growth at the

expense of sustained qualitative development (Tsouros and Farrington 2003).
Consequently a healthy city should foster an ecologically sound and secure local
environment, a diverse and equitable local economy, and a reduction in
inequalities leading to the social integration of diverse groups (ODPM 2003).
Individual and community awareness and responsibility are prerequisites for a
strong commitment by policy decision makers and practitioners to the re-
definition of goals and values that promote health and wellbeing in cities (WHO
1995). Without this commitment, based on a sound knowledge base and shared
goals and values, recent requests for more public participation cannot redefine
policy formulation and implementation in meaningful ways. Before individuals
and community groups can effectively participate with scientists, professionals
and politicians in policy formulation and implementation there are long-
standing institutional and social barriers that need to be addressed, as Lawrence
(1995) has argued. This implies very different approaches to mutual learning
from practitioners and has deeper implications for the education and training of
professionals and politicians.

9   *A form that is compatible with and enhances the preceding characteristics* of urban
areas points to twentieth-century urbanization transforming the physical, psychological and social dimensions of daily life including housing, transport and
other characteristics of metropolitan areas. For example, improved access to
medical services is a common characteristic of urban neighbourhoods that is rare
in rural areas. Urban life has other important health benefits including easy
access to job markets, education, cultural and leisure activities (Lawrence 1999).
There are many types of human settlement layouts, including linear and nodal,
compact and dispersed. The concentration of many kinds of human activities,
the built environment and the resident population has many ecological and
economic advantages compared with a more dispersed form of human settlement. In essence, a compact form of human settlement uses less arable land,
which is a precious non renewable resource for the sustenance of all ecosystems
(Wackernagel and Rees 1996). In addition, the compact human settlement has a
lower unit cost for most kinds of infrastructure and services such as roads,
drainage, piped water and sanitation (Commission for Environmental Cooperation 1996; Barton and Tsourou 2000). One of the most significant changes
in the layout and growth of cities during the twentieth century was the trend for
the development of dispersed suburbs, rather than compact neighbourhoods.
For example, the resident population of New York increased by only 5 per cent in
the last 25 years of the twentieth century, whereas the surface area of its built
environment increased by 61 per cent (Girardet 1999). This kind of urban and
suburban sprawl has many negative impacts, including the increased loss of
fertile agricultural land, the destruction of forests, and irreversible damage to
wetlands and coastal ecosystems. The dispersed form of urban development has
larger ecological, economic and social costs than the compact city and some of
these costs can have negative impacts on health and wellbeing (Barton and
Tsourou 2000). Therefore, trends that dominated urban development during the
twentieth century should be regulated more strictly by land use controls in order

to make urban living less dependent on the ecological resource base. Architects and urban planners can promote ecological efficiency in existing urban neighbourhoods by not agreeing to design new out-of-town shopping malls or housing estates that are not accessible using public transport (Dubé 2000). These peripheral developments on the outskirts of cities convert productive agricultural land and forests into new suburban sprawl that destroys both the ecological and the social fabric of human settlements. They also frequently create dependence on cars, thus isolating those who do not drive, notably children, the disabled, the aged and the poor.

10 *An optimum level of appropriate public healthcare services accessible to all* is a rallying call to national and local governments, sometimes with the private sector, to take full responsibility for the institutions, organizations and resources that are devoted to promote, sustain or restore health. A health system has important functions including the provision of services and the human, monetary and physical resources that make the delivery of these services possible (WHO 2000a). These resources can include any contribution whether in informal personal healthcare, or public or private professional health and medical services. The primary purpose of all services is to improve health by preventive or curative measures. A health system should not only strive to attain the highest average level of the health status of the population, but also, simultaneously, to reduce the differences between the health of individuals and groups. Healthcare systems have the important responsibility to ensure that people are treated equitably, in an affordable manner and in accordance with human rights. Poor municipal management has not relieved the inadequacy of the quantity or quality of water supplied to populations in urban areas. For example, the joint WHO/UNICEF monitoring programme estimates that in Asia and the Pacific region less than 65 per cent have water supplied and less than 40 per cent of all households in urban agglomerations have a sewage connection (WHO/UNICEF 2000). These deficiencies can be compounded by poor environmental management such as the conversion of water catchment areas, deforestation in the hinterlands around cities, pollution from industrial production and landfill dumps for the disposal of solid wastes. According to available information, 85 per cent of India's urban population has access to drinking water but only 20 per cent of the available drinking water meets health and safety standards.

11 *High health status* (high levels of positive health and low levels of disease) is challenging because twenty-first-century urban health can be characterized by relatively high levels of tuberculosis, respiratory and cardiovascular diseases, cancers, adult obesity and malnutrition, tobacco smoking, mental ill health, alcohol consumption and drug abuse, sexually transmitted diseases (including AIDS), as well as fear of crime, homicides, violence and accidental injury and death (Vlahov and Galea 2002). It is noteworthy that in the 1990s mental ill health was integrated into the aetiology of urban health, and that the promotion of both physical and mental health were accepted as a complementary goal for national and local policy makers and professionals (Parry-Jones and Quelquoz

1991). Increasingly, the achievement of high health status is being understood as involving policy changes in sectors other than health including employment, housing, transport and town planning. The bringing together of public health and sustainable development provides a creative opportunity for new policies that may counter the urban health concerns that characterize living in cities. Unfortunately, during the 1990s, a number of negative trends related to the provision of basic infrastructure and services were recorded by UNCHS Habitat and other organizations. In particular, per capita investment in basic urban services declined for a number of reasons including urban population growth, especially on the outskirts of cities; in addition, lack of security of tenure offered little incentive for residents to invest in services themselves (UNCHS 2001). These recent trends in investment in basic infrastructure and services need to be highlighted and challenged by all those who promote public health because they present a major obstacle to the building of healthier cities.

From principles to professional practice

The 11 principles about building healthy cities in specific localities need to be understood and applied using innovative empirical research and professional practice. This stems from the fact that many contributions that are meant to address health promotion and prevention have not been wholly successful, even though many urban planners, public health officers and medical practitioners are convinced they have the right answers. There is an urgent need for innovative approaches in many situations, such as the continuing failure of the wealthiest countries of the world to provide all citizens with secure employment, affordable housing and appropriate healthcare that meet at least minimal requirements. The failure of so called model housing estates and urban planning projects constructed in the 1960s and 1970s in numerous cities around the world, clearly shows that new ideas, working methods, objectives and criteria are needed (Lawrence 2004).

   Our incapacity to deal with the above mentioned problems is related to the complexity of dealing with urban health, to the compartmentalization of scientific and professional knowledge about urban ecosystems, to the bureaucratic division of responsibilities in cities, and to the increasing diversity of living conditions between various cities and within specific cities. In addition, the lack of effective collaboration between scientists, professionals and policy decision makers has led to an applicability gap in sectors that deal with urban planning, public health and many other sectors concerned with the construction and maintenance of cities. These shortcomings of mainstream scientific research and professional practice are not necessarily the result of a lack of political commitment, or financial resources, or viable propositions. They are, above all, the logical outcome of the narrow vision of so called experts who do not address fundamental issues but only topics isolated from their urban context. A number of obstacles need to be overcome, including:

- conceptual frameworks that do not recognize the pertinence of an ecological interpretation of urban health and living conditions;
- methodological contributions that value rational, quantified interpretations of

illness and disease at the expense of qualitative interpretations of health and wellbeing;
* poor use and management of human and natural ecosystems;
* segmentation and bureaucratization of professional knowledge and expertise often at the expense of the experience of lay people.

The health status of populations in specific urban areas is not only the result of many material and immaterial constituents but also the relationships between them. Hence, several concepts and methods need to be examined to understand the constituents and the relationships between them. For example, a constituent should not be isolated from the context in which it occurs. Instead, ecological approaches ought to be applied to understand both the constituents and the relationships between them (Lawrence 2001).

The distinction between biomedical models and ecological interpretations of health is fundamental for urban health (Lawrence 1999). The germ theory, for example, is an incomplete explanation of human illness and disease because it ignores the contribution of numerous physical and social dimensions of the environment that can affect health. Ecological interpretations maintain that the presence of a germ is a necessary but not a sufficient condition for an individual to become ill. They accept that some individuals become more susceptible to certain illnesses because of their differential exposure to numerous environmental, economic and social factors that can promote or be harmful to health and wellbeing. This interpretation does not ignore the influence of genetics, individual behaviour or primary healthcare. However, it maintains that, alone, these do not address possible relations between social problems and illness, especially inequalities, or positive social dimensions and health promotion by public education. The distinction between potential and actual health status can be the foundation for a new interpretation of urban health which includes the way ecological, economic, social, political and psychological factors transgress traditional disciplinary boundaries in order to address specific issues that may be pertinent only in precise situations. In essence, these traditional disciplinary boundaries need to be challenged. Only then can counter interpretations and new ways of intersectoral collaboration be implemented with effective outcomes.

In concluding it is important to note that the interrelations between housing, urban planning, health, social and environmental policies have been poorly articulated in practice (WHO 2000c, 2000d). However, it is crucial to acknowledge the important role of cities as localities for the management of resources and as the social context for diverse cultures and lifestyles. Although housing and land use policies have rarely been a high priority in the manifestos of governments, trends indicate that policies that prioritize social cohesion and the quality of life in cities and towns are becoming important components of political agendas.

The Healthy Cities project faces major challenges. Beyond its core concerns and key principles, it will need to address both the mitigation and adaptation responses to global climate change (Fudge and Antrobus 2002). Current and future concerns about the regional and local impacts of global climate change will be coupled with projected increases in the numbers of elderly people living more than 80 years. The growing imbalance between those employed persons providing services and a tax base, and retired and unemployed persons will need to be addressed. What the future healthy and sustainable city comprises and how it will be constructed and managed will undoubtedly be influenced by the public health agenda. The current priorities are linked to an urgent need for the definition of key principles for professional practice.

References

Barton, H. and Tsourou, C. (2000) Healthy Urban Planning. London: E & FN Spon.

Commission for Environmental Cooperation (CEC) (1996) *European Sustainable Cities, Report of the Expert Group on the Urban Environment.* Brussels: DGXI.

DETR (1999) *Towards an Urban Renaissance.* London: HMSO.

Dubé, P. (2000) Urban health: an urban planning perspective, *Reviews on Environmental Health,* 15: 249–65.

Duffy, H. (1995) *Competitive Cities: Succeeding in a Global Economy.* London: E & FN Spon.

Ekblad, S. (1993) Stressful environments and their effects on quality of life in Third World cities, Environment and Urbanization, 5(2): 125–34.

Fudge, C. (2003a) The demographic time bomb, *Urban Design Quarterly,* summer issue, 87: 28–32.

Fudge, C. (2003b) Health and sustainability gains from urban regeneration and development, in T. Takano (ed.) *Healthy Cities and Urban Policy Research.* London: E & FN Spon.

Fudge, C. (2004) Implementing sustainable futures in cities, in J. Orme *et al.* (eds) *Multi-disciplinary Public Health.* Milton Keynes: Open University Press.

Fudge, C. (2005) *Sustainable Urban Development in Sweden.* Stockholm: Swedish Research Council for Environment, Agricultural Sciences and Spatial Planning.

Fudge, C. and Antrobus, G. (2002) *Climate Change Research Scoping Paper, Report to MISTRA.* Stockholm: The Swedish Foundation for Environmental Research.

Fudge, C. and Rowe, J. (2000) *Implementing Sustainable Futures in Sweden.* Stockholm: Swedish Building Research Council.

Fudge, C. and Rowe, J. (2001) Ecological modernisation as a framework for sustainable development: a case study in Sweden, *Environment and Planning, A,* 33: 1527–46.

Gabe, J. and Williams, P. (1993) Women, crowding and mental health, in R. Burridge, and D. Ormandy (eds) *Unhealthy Housing: Research, Remedy and Reform.* London: E & FN Spon.

Girardet, H. (1999) *Creating Sustainable Cities.* Schumacher Briefings No. 2. Dartington, UK: Green Books.

Godinho, J. (2005) Public health in the former Soviet Union, in A. Scriven and G. Garman (eds) (2005) *Promoting Health: Global Perspectives.* Basingstoke: Palgrave Macmillan.

Goldstein, G. (2000) Healthy cities: overview of a WHO international program, *Reviews on Environmental Health,* 15: 207–14.

Gray, A. (2001) *Definitions of Crowding and the Effects of Crowding on Health: A Literature Review.* Wellington: The Ministry of Social Policy, Research Series Report 1.

Green, G., Acres, F. and Price, C. (2003) City health development planning, in A. Tsouros and F. Farrington (eds) *WHO Healthy Cities in Europe: A Compilation of Papers on Progress and Achievements.* Copenhagen: World Health Organization European Office for Europe.

Halpern, D. (1995) *Mental Health and the Built Environment.* London: Taylor & Francis.

Laverack, G. (2001) An identification and interpretation of the organisational aspects of community empowerment, *Community Development Journal,* 36(2): 40–52.

Laverack, G. (2004) *Health Promotion Practice: Power and Empowerment.* London: Sage.

Lawrence, R. (1995) Meeting the challenge: barriers to integrate cross-sectoral urban policies, in M. Rolén (ed.) *Urban Policies for an Environmentally Sustainable World*. The OECD-Sweden seminar on the ecological city, 1–3 June 1994. Stockholm: Swedish Council for Planning and Co-ordination of Research.

Lawrence, R. (1999) Urban health: an ecological perspective, *Reviews on Environmental Health*, 14: 1–10.

Lawrence, R. (2001) Human ecology, in M.K. Tolba (ed.) *Our Fragile World: Challenges and Opportunities for Sustainable Development*, Vol. 1. Oxford: EOLLS Publishers.

Lawrence, R. (2002) Inequalities in urban areas: innovative approaches to complex issues,. *Scandinavian Journal of Public Health*, supplement 59: 34–40.

Lawrence, R. (2004) Housing and health: from interdisciplinary principles to transdisciplinary research and practice. *Futures*, 36: 487–502.

Lee, K. (1999) Globalisation and the need for strong public health response, *European Journal of Public Health*, 9: 249–50.

Ludermir, A. and Harpham, T. (1998) Urbanization and mental health in Brazil: social and economic dimensions, *Health and Place*, 4: 223–32.

Marmot, M. and Wilkinson, R. (eds) (1999) *Social Determinants of Health*. Oxford: Oxford University Press.

McDaid, D. and Oliver, A. (2005) Inequalities in health: international patterns and trends, in A. Scriven and G. Garman (eds) *Promoting Health: Global Perspectives*. Basingstoke: Palgrave Macmillan.

Mitchell, J. (ed.) (1999) *Crucibles of Hazards: Mega-cities and Disasters in Transition*. Tokyo: United Nations University Press.

OPDM (2003) *Sustainable Communities: Building for the Future*. London: HMSO.

Parry-Jones, W. and Quelquoz, N. (eds) (1991) *Mental Health and Deviance in Inner Cities*. Geneva: World Health Organization, document no. WHO/MNH/PSF/91.1.

Pederson, R., Robertson, A. and de Zeeuw, H. (2000) Food, health and the urban environment, *Reviews on Environmental Health*, 15: 231–47.

Schwela, D. (2000) Air pollution and health in urban areas, *Reviews on Environmental Health*, 15: 13–42.

Scriven, A. (2007) Developing local alliance partnerships through community collaboration and participation, in S. Handsley *et al.* (eds) *Policy and Practice in Promoting Public Health*. London: Sage.

Tsouros, A. and Farrington, J. (eds) (2003) *WHO Healthy Cities in Europe: A Compilation of Papers on Progress and Achievements*. Copenhagen: World Health Organization European Office for Europe.

UN (United Nations) (1992) *United Nations Conference on Environment and Development (UNCED) the Earth Summit*. London: Regency Press.

UNCHS (United Nations Commission on Human Settlements) (1996) *An Urbanizing World: Global Report on Human Settlements 1996*. Oxford: Oxford University Press.

UNCHS (United Nations Commission on Human Settlements) (2001) *The State of the World's Cities*. Nairobi: United Nations Commission on Human Settlements, document HS/619/01[E].

Vlahov, D. and Galea, S. (2002) Urbanization, urbanicity, and health, *Journal of Urban Health: Bulletin of the New York Academy of Medicine*, 79: supplement 1, S1–12.

Wackernagel, M. and Rees, W. (1996) *Our Ecological Footprint: Reducing Human Impact on Earth*. Gabriola Island: New Society Publishers.

Werna, E., Harpham, T. and Goldstein, G. (1998) *Healthy City Projects in Developing Countries: An International Approach to Local Problems.* London: Earthscan.

Werna, E., Harpham, T., Blue, I. and Goldstein, G. (1999) From healthy city projects to healthy cities, *Environment and Urbanization*, 11: 27–39.

WHO (World Health Organization) (1986) *Ottawa Charter for Health Promotion.* Geneva: WHO.

WHO (World Health Organization) (1990) *Indoor Environment: Health Aspects of Air Quality, Thermal Environment, Light and Noise.* Geneva: WHO, document WHO/EHE/RUD/90.2.

WHO (World Health Organization) (1995) *Health in Social Development: WHO Position Paper.* Geneva: WHO, document WHO/DGH/95.1.

WHO (World Health Organization) (1997) *Health and Environment in Sustainable Development: Five Years After the Earth Summit.* Geneva: WHO, document WHO/EHG/97.8.

WHO (World Health Organization) (1998) *Health 21: Health for All Policy Framework for the European Union.* Copenhagen: WHO.

WHO (World Health Organization) (2000a) *The World Health Report 2000: Health Systems: Improving Performance.* Geneva: WHO.

WHO (World Health Organization) (2000b) *Nutrition for Health and Development.* Geneva: WHO, document WHO/NHD/00.6.

WHO (World Health Organization) (2000c) *Healthy Cities in Action: 5 Case-studies from Africa, Asia, Middle East and Latin America.* Geneva: WHO, document WHO/SDE/PHE/00.02.

WHO (World Health Organization) (2000d) *Transport, Environment and Health.* Copenhagen: WHO, European Series No. 89.

WHO (World Health Organization) (2002) *Community Participation in Local Health and Sustainable Development: Approaches and Techniques.* Copenhagen: WHO, European Sustainable Development and Health Series No. 4.

WHO (World Health Organization) (2005) *Commission on the Social Determinants of Health: Towards a Conceptual Framework for Analysis and Action on the Social Determinants of Health.* Geneva: WHO.

WHO/UNICEF (World Health Organization & UNICEF) (2000) *Global Water Supply and Sanitation Assessment 2000 Report.* Geneva: WHO & UNICEF.

Wilkinson, R. (1996) *Unhealthy Societies: The Afflictions of Inequality.* London: Routledge.

17 From self-regulation to legislation: the social impact of public health action on smoking

Amanda Amos

Cigarette smoking is highly socially patterned. In countries which have the longest history of widespread smoking, such as the UK and USA, smoking is now strongly associated with social and material disadvantage. This reflects the history of the spread of the smoking epidemic around the world (Lopez *et al.* 1994). In the first decades of the twentieth century UK smokers were more likely to be affluent. Over recent decades this pattern has changed, reflecting lower uptake and higher cessation rates in affluent compared to disadvantaged groups. Today the highest smoking rates are among people who have low socioeconomic status, low educational attainment, low income, live in areas of deprivation and are socially marginalized (such as prisoners and people with mental health problems). For example, in 2004 in Britain 31 per cent of men in manual groups smoked compared with 22 per cent in non manual groups (Goddard and Green 2005). Smoking is now the most important cause of both preventable illness and death and inequalities in health, accounting for half the difference in survival to age 70 between socioeconomic groups I and V (Wanless 2004). There has also been a major change in the gender patterning of smoking. Women took up smoking in large numbers several decades after men and then had a slower decline in prevalence. Since the peak of smoking in the UK in the 1970s, the gap between men's and women's smoking has narrowed (see Figure 17.1). In 2004, 26 per cent of men and 23 per cent of women smoked. Among 12–15 year olds the rate of smoking among girls is now greater than among boys. In Scotland in 2004, 24 per cent of 15-year-old girls were regular smokers compared with 14 per cent of boys (CAHRU 2005).

Awareness about the increasing association between smoking and disadvantage started to emerge in the 1980s (Jacobson 1981; Graham 1987). However, it is only in the last few years that this relationship and its importance in reducing inequalities in health have received serious attention at the policy level and action has started to be taken to address this. In this chapter, there will be a brief outline of the evolution of different approaches to tobacco control in the UK. Key elements of current tobacco control policies at the national and international levels will be described and their impact considered, particularly in relation to reducing inequalities and smoking. Finally some challenges for the future will be highlighted.

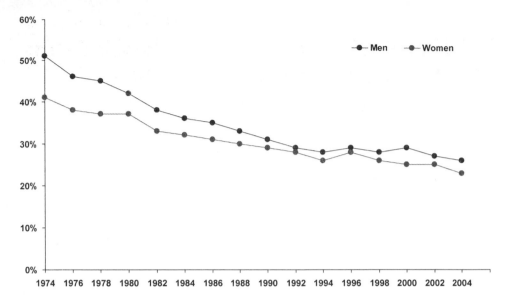

Figure 17.1 Prevalence of cigarette smoking in Great Britain by sex, adults aged 16 and over
Source: Goddard and Green (2005)

Smoker heal thyself

Until the 1980s smoking was generally constructed and addressed as a problem located within the individual. Reflecting the dominance at the time of the medical model and the preventive/behavioural model of health education (Ewles and Simnett 2003), the focus was on persuasion and education. The underlying assumption was that smoking was a lifestyle choice and thus if young people were informed about the risks they would be inoculated against becoming smokers. Similarly it was expected that smokers when made aware of the major risks to their health would quit. Public health attention focused on hard hitting media campaigns (mostly directed at men) and encouraging doctors to advise their patients to quit (Russell *et al.* 1979; Amos and Ineson 1989; Amos 1993).

Increasing public awareness of the risks of smoking did impact on smoking behaviour, with male cigarette smoking declining from 51 per cent in 1974 to 36 per cent in 1984 (see Figure 17.1). But the decline over this period was much less in women, from 41 per cent to 32 per cent, and the gap between advantaged and disadvantaged smokers increased. While over 40 per cent of socioeconomic group I smokers quit between 1974 and 1984, less than 20 per cent of socioeconomic group V smokers quit. Thus, as has been found consistently for a range of health-related behaviours, individualistic predominantly educational victim-blaming approaches (see Chapter 11 for further discussion of victim blaming) proved more effective in affluent advantaged groups (Ewles and Simnett 2003). With reference to the classic epidemiological triangle of disease causation most attention was focused on the host (the smoker or potential smoker) with little attention being given to either the agent of disease (cigarettes/tobacco) or environmental factors (such as socioeconomic circumstances or the tobacco industry).

Lobbying by the group Action on Smoking and Health (ASH) and medical organizations including the Royal College of Physicians (RCP) and the British Medical Association (BMA) did eventually lead the then Conservative government to acknowledge that smoking was the biggest preventable cause of ill health, but did not succeed in persuading it to significantly limit the freedom of the tobacco industry to produce, promote and sell cigarettes. Action was limited to placing health warnings (including tar content) on products and advertising, and weak voluntary restrictions on promotion. Smoking, like other behavioural risk factors such as diet and alcohol consumption, continued to be seen as a matter of individual choice (DHSS 1976; Amos and Ineson 1989). The socioeconomic and gender distribution of these issues was raised only to berate groups of people, including the working class, nurses and northerners, about their appalling health behaviours (Carvel 1987; Lyall 1987).

The 1980s and 1990s saw increasing calls to address the wider determinants of smoking, including the activities of the tobacco industry and social and cultural factors, as concern mounted about the levelling off of the decline in adult smoking and the increasing inequalities gap (see Figure 17.1). A growing body of research was starting to generate new insights about the relationship between smoking and inequalities, including the importance of the social context of smoking (Graham 1993; Marsh and McKay 1994), as well of the influence of tobacco companies' activities including marketing. The emergence of health promotion and the new public health (see Chapter 2 for further examination of the new public health) at the local, national and international levels, with their focus on equity and the politics of health, led to increased lobbying on this issue and the development of innovative approaches focusing on inequalities such as exploring community based, bottom-up initiatives on smoking in disadvantaged communities (Gaunt-Richardson *et al.* 1999; Ritchie *et al.* 2004). The emergence of new cost effective pharmacotherapies that produced higher quit rates than advice alone renewed interest in providing cessation support more widely. At the same time an international consensus was emerging about the key elements of a comprehensive tobacco control strategy and a need for a global approach.

Government action, however, remained limited. While the government had become convinced about the impact of price on cigarette consumption (and that increasing tax also increased revenue), and had regularly increased tax on cigarettes, resisted taking substantive action to control tobacco companies (such as banning tobacco promotion), other than that required by European (EU) directives on market harmonization. Targets were set to reduce smoking but action to achieve them still focused primarily on education with no account of social determinants (DoH 1992; Scottish Office 1992).

Smoking kills: a comprehensive approach

The election of the Labour government in 1997 proved a milestone in tobacco control. Not only because it promised to tackle the tobacco industry, most notably by banning tobacco advertising, but it was the first government to frame smoking as an inequalities and health issue. In 1998 it became the first British government to adopt a comprehensive tobacco control strategy. The White Paper *Smoking Kills* (DoH 1998) set out action to be taken over the following three years to tackle smoking prevention and cessation (see Table 17.1).

Table 17.1   Key elements of the UK government's 1998 White Paper on tobacco

Protecting children and young people
- Minimal tobacco advertising in shops
- Tough enforcement on underage sales
- Proof of age card
- Strong rules on siting of cigarette vending machines

Smoking and adults
- Over £60 million to be spent on new NHS services to help people stop smoking, starting in the most deprived areas
- GPs will be able to refer people who want to quit for specialist advice and, for those least able to afford to buy it, one week's free nicotine replacement therapy
- Pregnant women who smoke will be a priority

Tobacco advertising and promotion
- Legislation to end tobacco advertising and sponsorship
- Ban to be phased in with global sports, such as Formula One racing, having the longest period

Changing attitudes
- £50 million to be spent over next three years on a major new media campaign on tobacco

Drive against smuggling
- £35 million package of measures to tackle alcohol and tobacco smuggling, to reduce £1 billion a year lost through tobacco smuggling

Clean air and smoking at work
- People have a right to be protected against smoking. Will not ban smoking in public places but agree a new charter on smoking with the licensed trade
- Not banning smoking at work, but will consult on a new Approved Code of Practice on smoking at work

Taxation
- Increase tobacco taxation by an average of 5 per cent in real terms each year

Smoking and international action
- Opposes harmonization of taxes across EU but wants to increase the minimum levels of tobacco duty in the EU
- Will support world health campaigns and the development of a new international convention on tobacco control

Source: Department of Health (1998)

While some of the strategy re-endorsed previous policies (for example prevention of sales to children, media campaigns, taxation) albeit with extra funding and support, it also included more radical action to support smokers who wanted to quit, ban tobacco promotion, tackle tobacco smuggling and support international action. However, the strategy stopped far short of banning smoking in public places. Rather the government committed itself to progressing voluntary agreements with the licensed trade and employers.

Smoking Kills marked a step change in the political priority, the breadth of the approach and the level of investment in tackling smoking. The White Paper included five of the six policies identified by the World Bank as cost-effective and which should be prioritized in tobacco control programmes (see Table 17.2).

Table 17.2 Cost-effective interventions in tobacco control

- Higher taxes on cigarettes and other tobacco products
- Bans/restrictions on smoking in public and workplaces
- Comprehensive bans on advertising and promotion of all tobacco products, logos and brand names
- Better consumer information
- Large, direct warning labels on cigarette packs and other tobacco products
- Help for smokers who wish to quit, including increased access to NRT and other cessation therapies

Source: World Bank (2003)

Furthermore the original three-year strategy has continued to be supported and developed by government – for example, in England through the public health White Paper *Choosing Health* (DoH 2004a) and in Scotland through its own national tobacco control action plan *A Breath of Fresh Air* (Scottish Executive 2004). Increased funding has been provided for local smoking cessation services and media campaigns (particularly on the health effects of second-hand smoke), and smoking targets have been revised (DoH 2004a, 2004b). A recent analysis of national tobacco control policies in 30 countries in Europe in 2005, using a scale based on the World Bank recommended actions, ranked the UK second after Ireland, gaining 73 out of a maximum 100 points (Joossens and Raw 2006).

This strategy appears to be reducing adult smoking. After little decline in adult smoking rates in Britain during the 1990s, between 2000 and 2004 male smoking declined from 29 per cent to 26 per cent and from 25 to 23 per cent in women. However there appears to have been less of an impact on young people. Between 2000 and 2005 regular smoking among 11–15-year-olds in England declined only from 10 to 9 per cent (NCSR 2006). Regular smoking among 15 year olds decreased from 23 to 20 per cent but most of this decline was in boys (21 to 16 per cent) with little change in girls (26 to 25 per cent). In Scotland there was little change in regular smoking between 2000 and 2004 in boys (15 to 14 per cent) and none in girls (24 per cent) (CAHRU 2005). In response to these figures the Scottish health minister convened a working group on smoking prevention in young people to advise on what action should be taken (Smoking Prevention Working Group 2006).

Smoking Kills was also groundbreaking in clearly stating the government's aim to reduce inequalities in smoking. Smokers living on low incomes were identified as one of the three priority groups, along with young people and pregnant women. Subsequently national smoking inequalities targets have been set. In England the target is to reduce smoking rates among manual groups from 32 per cent in 1998 to 26 per cent in 2010 (DoH 2000). In Scotland the targets focus on reducing smoking in the most deprived area quintile, from 37.3 per cent in 2004 to 33.2 per cent in 2008 in adults and among pregnant women from 35.8 per cent in 2003 to 32.2 per cent in 2008 (www.clearing theairscotland.com). In 2004 cigarette smoking in manual groups in England declined to 30 per cent (Goddard and Green 2005). However, since the prevalence of smokers in non-manual groups declined by a similar amount (22 per cent in 1998 to 20 per cent in 2004) there was no significant reduction in the gap between these groups. This raises a key question: are current tobacco control policies in the UK likely to reduce inequalities in smoking, or has there been a failure to address this challenge in the pursuit of reducing overall tobacco consumption, as found in other countries (Platt *et al.* 2002)? The next part of the chapter will address this question by considering the six key strands of current national policies and their likely impact on disadvantaged smokers.

UK tobacco control: reducing inequalities and smoking?

Raising tobacco taxes and tackling smuggling

The price of cigarettes and tobacco is the single most important determinant of levels of consumption (World Bank 2003). Higher taxes reduce adult cigarette consumption (though not prevalence) and smoking uptake among young people. A 10 per cent increase in cigarette price on average reduces demand in adults by 4 per cent and has an even greater impact on young people's consumption (Jha and Chaloupka 1999). There is also evidence that in high-income countries like the UK tobacco tax increases reduce consumption disproportionately among low socioeconomic groups. Thus regular above inflation increases in tobacco tax, as promised in *Smoking Kills*, should impact more on smoking among disadvantaged groups. However it has been argued that this policy is regressive as it hits hardest those on low incomes who find it most difficult to quit. While this view has been challenged (Warner 2000), concern has been expressed that this policy ignores the personal and material dimensions of disadvantage that bind people to smoking. The government has argued that this is addressed through other tobacco control policy strands, notably providing free cessation support, as well as through social and welfare policies aimed at reducing social exclusion and poverty. A more direct way of addressing this concern would be to hypothecate a proportion of tax revenues to reducing the social determinants of smoking. In the 2000 Budget the Chancellor of the Exchequer raised cigarette taxes by 5 per cent above inflation, stating that some of the money accruing from this increase would go to the National Health Service (NHS). The Scottish Executive received £26 million, which it invested in a major health improvement programme aimed at reducing inequalities. However these tax increases have not been sustained. The 2004 Budget tobacco duty rates were only in line with inflation and the 2006 increase was lower than inflation. As a result cigarettes have become cheaper in real terms, thus negating any impact on consumption.

The 1990s saw a massive increase in the smuggling of tobacco and cigarettes. By 1999 25–33 per cent of all tobacco products smoked in the UK were smuggled or contraband. There is clear evidence that tobacco companies were complicit in smuggling (Joossens and Raw 1998, 2000; ASH 2004). Smuggled tobacco products are particularly prevalent in deprived areas and thus may have a disproportionate impact on smoking behaviour and attitudes in these communities (Wiltshire *et al.* 2001). Cheap smuggled cigarettes and tobacco undermine the impact of government policies on price. The increased investment in tackling smuggling had significantly reduced the market to around 18 per cent in 2003, but an increasing proportion of smuggled cigarettes are counterfeit and are even more damaging to health. In 2006 tobacco smuggling still cost an estimated £2.5 billion a year in lost tax revenue (HM Treasury 2006).

Smoking cessation services

One of the most important and innovative element of *Smoking Kills* was the establishment of the NHS Stop Smoking Services. The UK is the first country in the world to provide nationwide local specialist cessation services (McNeill *et al.* 2005). These aim to provide evidence based support to the 70 per cent of smokers who want to quit. This involves offering individual or group support combined with pharmacotherapies, usually nicotine replacement therapy (NRT) or Zyban. Clinical trials have shown that combining pharmacotherapy and support increases one-year quit rates to 15–20 per cent, four times the unaided rate (West *et al.* 2000). There is also a focus on targeting the services to disadvantaged groups. The English services were initially established in Health Action Zones (HAZs) (areas with poorest health; see Chapter 12 for a detailed evaluation of HAZs) before being rolled out. NRT and Zyban are also available on prescription and thus free to smokers on benefits. In addition there are telephone helplines for smokers, pregnant smokers and different ethnic groups.

Local services were used by over 500,000 smokers in 2004/5 and in England achieved quit rates comparable to clinical trials (Ferguson *et al.* 2005). Previous studies of smoking cessation services found that low-income smokers were less likely to use cessation services and that their quit rates were lower than those of more affluent smokers (Richardson 2001). Indeed nicotine addiction increases systematically with deprivation. This poses challenges for cessation services in terms of how they can become more attractive and accessible to disadvantaged smokers, and the nature of the support they offer. The findings from the evaluation of the English services have been positive, indicating that in their first couple of years they reached proportionally more smokers from disadvantaged areas, though they had lower quit rates than smokers from more prosperous areas (Judge and Bauld 2004). Overall these services probably contributed to reducing inequalities in smoking. However, while these treatment services are highly cost-effective, their impact on reducing smoking prevalence will be small, around 0.5–1.0 per cent a year, and on their own would take several decades to reduce inequalities in smoking (Judge and Bauld 2004; Wanless 2004).

Reducing tobacco advertising and promotion

Following a European Directive, tobacco advertising was banned in the UK and the EU in 2002 and tobacco sponsorship was banned in 2005. Comprehensive national bans on tobacco promotion, including advertising and other forms of marketing such as sponsorship, have been shown to reduce smoking prevalence, including uptake in young people (Saffer and Chaloupka 2000). The World Bank estimates that comprehensive bans can reduce tobacco consumption by around 7 per cent (Jha and Chaloupka 1999). It is not known whether such bans have a differential effect on disadvantaged groups and the impact of the ban in the UK is not yet clear. However, there is evidence that tobacco companies have targeted deprived areas and low socioeconomic groups and thus they are likely to benefit most from bans (Kunst *et al.* 2004). However, tobacco is still marketed in the UK through a variety of media and promotional devices. For example, cigarettes are still displayed prominently in thousands of shops. Positive images of smokers, including celebrities, continue to be shown in films, TV and magazines, including youth magazines, and these images are particularly salient for young people (MacFadyen *et al.* 2003; Charlesworth and Glantz 2005).

Regulating tobacco products

There are several European Directives regulating tobacco products which the UK has implemented. These include limiting the tar content of cigarettes, banning misleading descriptors such as 'light' and 'mild', and requiring large direct health warnings on tobacco products (ASPECT 2005). Hard-hitting pictorial warnings are due to appear on cigarette packs in 2007. Large health warnings increase public awareness of the health effects of smoking, discouraging smoking, and move smokers towards quitting (Hammond *et al.* 2004; ASPECT 2005). However, it is not known if these measures contribute to reducing inequalities in smoking. One new proposal is to require cigarettes to have reduced ignition propensity in order to avoid fires, as is already required in parts of the USA (Connolly *et al.* 2005). Cigarettes are the main cause of fires in the UK, and this measure would significantly reduce deaths and injuries from fires, particulary in low-income households (ASH 2006).

Media campaigns

Sustained and well-funded media campaigns as part of comprehensive tobacco control programmes can increase adult smokers' motivation to quit and reduce smoking (World Bank 2003). In the UK mass media campaigns increase calls to telephone quitlines and are more effective in reaching disadvantaged smokers (Platt *et al.* 1997; Stead *et al.* 2003). There is also some, though weak, evidence that media campaigns can reduce smoking uptake in young people (Sowden and Arblaster 1998). Youth-oriented campaigns have a poor record of credibility with young people and can risk reinforcing rather than discouraging smoking (see www.hbi.de/help-eu/pdfs/Commission_leaflet.pdf). However, some recent campaigns have developed innovative approaches that engage youth in ways and on issues that they find salient and credible. For example, the Truth campaigns in the USA, which have focused on the tobacco industry's deceitful marketing practices (Hersey *et al.* 2005). Campaigns aimed at adults can also be effective in reaching young people and help discredit the aspirational adult image of smoking. Media campaigns can play an important role in increasing awareness about the risks of passive smoking, thereby increasing support for the introduction and implementation of smoke free legislation. This may be particularly important for disadvantaged families and communities who have fewer restrictions on smoking in their local bars and pubs (Plunkett *et al.* 2000) and in their homes (Scottish Executive 2005).

Reducing exposure to second-hand smoke

Exposure to second hand smoke (SHS) is a significant cause of premature mortality and morbidity, causing at least 10,000 deaths a year in the UK (Hole 2004; Jamrozik 2005). Growing awareness of the health effects has led to increasing restrictions on smoking in public places, notably workplaces. Several countries (Ireland, Italy, Norway, New Zealand), and many states and cities in the USA and Australia have passed comprehensive legislation eliminating smoking in most enclosed (indoor) public places and many more are planning to do so. Comprehensive legislation not only results in significant reductions in SHS exposure, particularly in workplaces and leisure facilities such as bars

(Allwright *et al.* 2005), and mortality (Ludbrook *et al.* 2004), but can have potentially even more important public health benefits by reducing smoking and changing social attitudes and norms about smoking. Workplace bans have shown associated declines in consumption, increased attempts to quit and increased rates of successful quitting (Fichtenberg and Glantz 2002; Ludbrook *et al.* 2004). Smoking bans can affect smoking-related attitudes that influence smoking uptake and cessation, notably the perceived prevalence of smoking and perceived social acceptability of smoking in the community (Albers *et al.* 2004). Such legislation is likely to have more impact in disadvantaged than affluent communities. Not only is smoking more prevalent in these communities but local bars and pubs are less likely to have smoking policies (Plunkett *et al.* 2000).

The UK government has been disappointingly slow in taking effective action on this issue. While *Smoking Kills* recognized that reducing exposure to SHS was important, action was restricted to encouraging workplaces and others to take voluntary action. Despite increasing evidence on the risks to health, the limited voluntary action (only 50 per cent of workplaces were smoke free in 2003) and the comprehensive legislation being implemented elsewhere, as recently as 2004, the UK government's policy remained one of encouraging employers and others to ensure that smoke-free becomes the norm (DoH 2004a). For this element of tobacco control it appeared that individual choice remained the government's overriding imperative, as exemplified by the then British Health Minister, Dr John Reid, arguing for freedom of choice and not denying poor people their only pleasure. This policy was widely criticized by those within tobacco control and public health more generally. Indeed the English Chief Medical Officer Sir Liam Donaldson considered resigning over the government's position. Most critics pointed out that comprehensive legislation would reduce not only SHS but also smoking and that this would have most impact in disadvantaged communities, thereby helping to reduce inequalities in smoking. It was therefore perhaps not surprising that Scotland, the part of the UK where smoking has the greatest impact on inequalities in health, decided to take its own action on this issue (ASH Scotland 2005). On 26 March 2006 the Scottish Executive implemented its comprehensive legislation on the prohibition of smoking in enclosed public places (www.clearingtheairscotland.com). In striking contrast to the UK government's position, the Scottish First Minister, Jack McConnell, described this as the most important public health legislation in a generation. In spring 2006, following enormous public pressure on the UK government, legislation was passed which should produce a comprehensive ban in England, Wales and Northern Ireland. However, at the time of writing discussions are continuing as to possible exemptions including private clubs.

One continuing concern is that smoke free legislation might result in the displacement of smoking from public to private (homes, cars) spaces, thereby increasing SHS exposure in families including children. This might impact more on disadvantaged families. For example, in 2004 fewer than half of homes in Scotland had total smoking bans and these were more common in middle class homes (Scottish Executive 2005); 40 per cent of 8-15 year-olds lived in households where at least one person regularly smoked inside. Thus a shift in smoking to homes could exacerbate health inequalities by increasing disadvantaged children's exposure to SHS. However, there is no evidence that smoke free public places increase children's exposure to SHS at home (RCP 2005). Rather, research on the impact of bans in California and Australia suggests that there are associated increases in restrictions in the home (Borland *et al.* 1999; Gilpin *et al.* 2002).

As we move into the twenty first century it would appear that national tobacco control policies in the UK are at last starting to take serious account of the social determinants of smoking, perhaps more than any other country (Platt *et al.* 2002). However, significant challenges remain, as there has been little reduction in the gap between the smoking rates in the most and least affluent groups. Providing smoking cessation services is important, but while there has been some success at reaching disadvantaged smokers, little progress has been made in increasing their effectiveness in helping them to quit. There is a need to test new models of cessation support – for example, providing services that are more intensive, flexible, that include relapse prevention and are community based. But even with increased levels of effectiveness and funding, cessation services can have only a limited impact at the population level. In addition, little progress has been made in reducing smoking uptake among young people.

The UK, with Ireland, has the most comprehensive tobacco control policies in Europe, but this is no cause for complacency. Achieving more rapid reductions in smoking is possible, as shown by Australia and US states like California and Massachusetts, where smoking rates are now considerably lower than in the UK. These have invested significantly higher levels of funding in comprehensive tobacco control. However, the challenge remains as to how to increase the equity impact of tobacco control strategies, a challenge that no country has successfully addressed. It also means addressing the wider social determinants of smoking, not least disadvantage, poverty and exclusion, which over the life course act both as pathways into smoking and barriers to quitting (INWAT Europe 2000; Bostock 2003).

For the UK, which has some of the most successful tobacco companies in the world (British American Tobacco controls 17 per cent of the world's tobacco market), this also means ensuring that reducing smoking at home does not result in tobacco companies pushing their lethal products even more strongly to growing markets in developing countries, thereby increasing global inequalities in health. It is essential that the UK government maintains its commitment to supporting international action on tobacco control. This includes supporting the wider ratification and implementation of the Framework Convention on Tobacco Control, the first global public health treaty negotiated under the auspices of the World Health Organization (WHO) (WHO 2005). This was adopted by the WHO member countries in 2003 and has been ratified by over 120 countries and the EU, who now have to implement it. It also means addressing international trade policies that prioritize the rights of corporations, and thus the tobacco industry, over health and human rights, and thereby threaten existing tobacco control policies and restrict the possibility of implementing new controls (Shaffer *et al.* 2005).

References

Albers, A.B., Siegal, M., Cheng, D.M., Biener, L. and Rigotti, N.A. (2004) Relation between local restaurant smoking regulations and attitudes towards the prevalence and social acceptability of smoking, *Tobacco Control*, 13: 347–55.

Allwright, S., Paul, G., Greiner, B., Mullally, B.J., Pursell, L., Kelly, A., Bonner, B., D'Eath, M., McConnell, B., McLaughlin, J.P., O'Donovan, D., O'Kane, E. and Perry, I.J. (2005)

Legislation for smoke-free workplaces and health of bar workers in Ireland: before and after study, *British Medical Journal*, 331: 1117–20.

Amos, A. (1993) In her own best interests? Women and health education – a review of the last 50 years, *Health Education Journal*, 50: 140–50.

Amos, A. and Ineson, A. (1989) Beyond individual choice – tobacco in the public health movement, in C.J. Martin and D.V. McQueen (eds) *Readings for a New Public Health*. Edinburgh: Edinburgh University Press.

ASH (2004) *Tobacco Smuggling.* Factsheet 17, www.ash.org.uk/html/factsheets/html/fact17.html.

ASH (2006) *Smoking Kills – Setting a Standard for the EU. Briefing Document.* London: ASH.

ASH Scotland (2005) *The Unwelcome Guest: How Scotland Invited the Tobacco Industry to Smoke Outside.* Edinburgh: ASH Scotland.

ASPECT (2005) *Tobacco or Health in the European Union: Past, Present and Future*, www.eu.int/comm/health/ph_determinants/life_style/Tobacco/Documents/tobacco_fr_en.pdf.

Borland, R., Mullins, R., Trotter, L. and White, V. (1999) Trends in environmental tobacco smoke restrictions in the home in Victoria, Australia, *Tobacco Control*, 8: 266–71.

Bostock, Y. (2003) *Searching for the Solution: Women, Smoking and Inequalities in Europe.* London: HDA/INWAT.

CAHRU (Child and Adolescent Health Research Unit) (2005) *Scottish Schools Adolescent Lifestyle and Substance use Survey (SALSUS) – National Report 2004.* Edinburgh: TSO.

Carvel, J. (1987) Commons debate on health promotion, *The Lancet*, 1037–8.

Charlesworth, A. and Glantz, S.A. (2005) Smoking in the movies increases adolescents smoking: a review, *Paediatrics*, 116: 1516–28.

Connolly, G.N., Alpert, G.R., Rees, V., Carpenter, C. and Wayne, G.F. (2005) Effect of the New York State cigarette fire safety standard on ignition propensity, smoke constituents, and the consumer market, *Tobacco Control*, 4: 321–7.

DHSS (Department of Health and Social Services) (1976) *Prevention and Health: Everybody's Business.* London: HMSO.

DoH (Department of Health) (1992) *The Health of the Nation: A Strategy for Health in England.* London: HMSO.

DoH (Department of Health) (1998) *Smoking Kills – A White Paper on Tobacco.* London: TSO.

DoH (Department of Health) (2000) *NHS Cancer Plan.* London: TSO.

DoH (Department of Health) (2004a) *Choosing Health – Making Healthier Choices Easier.* London: TSO.

DoH (Department of Health) (2004b) *Spending Review Public Service Agreements.* London: TSO.

Ewles, L. and Simnett, I. (2003) *Promoting Health – A Practical Guide.* Edinburgh: Bailliere Tindall.

Ferguson, J., Bauld, L., Chesterman, J. and Judge, K. (2005) The English smoking treatment services: one-year outcomes, *Addiction*, 100(Suppl. 2): s1–11.

Fichtenberg, C.M. and Glantz, S.A. (2002) Effect of smoke-free workplaces on smoking behaviour: systematic review, *British Medical Journal*, 325: 188–91.

Gaunt-Richardson, P., Amos, A., Howie, G,. McKie, L. and Moore, M. (1999) *Women, Low Income and Smoking: Breaking Down the Barriers.* Edinburgh: ASH Scotland/HEBS.

Gilpin, E.A., Farkas, A.J., Emery, S.L., Ake, C.F. and Pierce, J.P. (2002) Clean indoor air: advances in California, 1990–1999, *American Journal of Public Health*, 92: 785–91.

Goddard, E. and Green, H. (2005) *Smoking and Drinking among Adults, 2004. General Household Survey 2004.* London: ONS.

Graham, H. (1987) Women's smoking and family health, *Social Science and Medicine,* 25: 47–56.

Graham, H. (1993) *When Life's A Drag: Women, Smoking and Disadvantage.* London: HMSO.

Hammond, D., Fong, G.T., McDonald, P.W., Brown, K.S. and Cameron R. (2004) Graphic Canadian cigarette warning labels and adverse outcomes: evidence from Canadian smokers, *American Journal of Public Health,* 94: 1443–5.

Hersey, J.C., Niederdeppe, J., Ng, S.W., Mowery, P., Farrelly, M. and Messeri, P. (2005) How state counter-industry campaigns help prime perceptions of tobacco industry practices to promote reductions in youth smoking, *Tobacco Control,* 14: 377–83.

HM Treasury (2006) *Budget 2006. A Strong and Strengthening Economy: Investing in Britain's Future* www.hm-treasury.gov.uk/budget/budget_06/budget_report/bud_bud06_repindex.cfm.

Hole, D. (2004) *Passive Smoking and Associated Causes of Death in Adults in Scotland.* Edinburgh: NHS Health Scotland.

INWAT Europe (2000) *Part of the Solution? Tobacco Control Policies and Women.* London: HDA.

Jacobson, B. (1981) *The Ladykillers: Why Smoking is a Feminist Issue.* London: Pluto Press.

Jamrozik, K. (2005) Estimate of deaths attributable to passive smoking among UK adults: database analysis, *British Medical Journal,* doi:10.1136/bmj.38370.496632.8F.

Jha, P. and Chaloupka, F.J. (1999) *Curbing the Epidemic: Governments and the Economics of Tobacco Control.* Washington, DC: World Bank.

Joossens, L. and Raw, M. (1998) Cigarette smuggling in Europe: who really benefits? *Tobacco Control,* 7: 66–71.

Joossens, L. and Raw, M. (2000) How can cigarette smuggling be reduced? *British Medical Journal,* 321: 947–50.

Joossens, L. and Raw, M. (2006) The tobacco control scale: a new scale to measure country activity, *Tobacco Control,* 15: 247–53.

Judge, K. and Bauld, L. (2004) *NHS Stop Smoking Services and Health Inequalities in England.* Paper presented at the Faculty of Public Health annual conference, Edinburgh.

Kunst, A., Giskes, K. and Mackenbach, J. (2004) *Socioeconomic Inequalities in Smoking in the European Union.* Brussels: European Network for Smoking Prevention.

Lopez, A.D., Collishaw, N.E. and Piha, T. (1994) A descriptive model of the cigarette epidemic in developed countries, *Tobacco Control,* 3: 242–7.

Ludbrook, A., Bird, S. and van Teijlingen, E. (2004) *International Review of the Health and Economic Impact of the Regulation of Smoking in Public Places.* Edinburgh: NHS Health Scotland.

Lyall, J. (1987) Nurses' lifestyle attacked, *Health Services Journal,* 13 November: 1305.

MacFadyen, L., Amos, A., Hastings, G. and Parkes, E. (2003) 'They look like my kind of people'– perceptions of smoking images in youth magazines, *Social Science and Medicine,* 56: 491–9.

McNeill, A., Raw, M., Whybrow, J. and Bailey, P. (2005) A national strategy for smoking cessation treatment in England, *Addiction,* 100(Suppl. 2): s1–11.

Marsh, A. and McKay, S. (1994) *Poor Smokers.* London: PSI.

NCSR (National Center for Social Research) (2006) *Drug Use, Smoking and Drinking among Young People in England in 2005.* London: NHS, HSCIS.

Platt, S., Tannahill, A., Watson, J. and Fraser, E. (1997) Effectiveness of antismoking telephone helpline: follow up survey, *British Medical Journal,* 314: 1371–5.

Platt, S., Amos, A., Gnich, W. and Parry, O. (2002) Smoking policies, in J. Mackenbach and M. Bakker (eds) *Reducing Inequalities in Health: A European Perspective*. London: Routledge.

Plunkett, M., Haw, S., Cassels, J., Moore, M. and O'Connor, M. (2000) *Smoking in Public Places – A Survey of the Scottish Leisure Industry*. Edinburgh: ASH Scotland/HEBS.

RCP (Royal College of Physicians) (2005) *Going Smoke-free – The Medical Case for Clean Air in the Home, at Work and in Public Places*. London: RCP.

Richardson, K. (2001) *Smoking, Low Income and Health Inequalities*. London: ASH/HDA.

Ritchie, D., Parry, O., Gnich, W. and Platt, S. (2004) Issues of participation, ownership and empowerment in a community development programme: tackling smoking in a low-income area in Scotland, *Health Promotion International*, 9: 51–9.

Russell, M.A., Wilson, C. and Taylor, C. (1979) Effect of general practitioners' advice against smoking, *British Medical Journal*, ii: 231–5.

Saffer, H. and Chaloupka, F. (2000) The effect of tobacco advertising bans on tobacco consumption, *Journal of Health Economics*, 19: 1117–37.

Scottish Executive (2004) *A Breath of Fresh Air for Scotland: Improving Scotland's Health – the Challenge*. Edinburgh: Scottish Executive.

Scottish Executive (2005) *Smoking in Public Places: November 2005 Omnibus Survey Report*, www.smokefreescotland.com.

Scottish Office (1992) *Scotland's Health: A Challenge to Us All*. Edinburgh: HMSO.

Scottish Prevention Working Group (2006) *Towards a Future Without Tobacco*. Edinburgh: Scottish Executive.

Shaffer, E.R., Brenner, J.E. and Houston, T.P. (2005) International trade agreements: a threat to tobacco control policy, *Tobacco Control*, 14(Suppl. II): ii19–25.

Sowden, A.J. and Arblaster, L. (1998) Mass media interventions for preventing smoking in young people, *Cochrane Database of Systematic Reviews*, 4.

Stead, L., Lancaster, T. and Perera, R. (2003) *Telephone Counselling for Smoking Cessation*. The Cochrane Library, Issue 1.

Wanless, D. (2004) *Securing Good Health for the Whole Population*. London: HM Treasury/DoH.

Warner, K.E. (2000) The economics of tobacco: myths and realities, *Tobacco Control*, 9: 78–89.

West, R., McNeill, A. and Raw, M. (2000) National smoking cessation guidelines for health professionals: an update. *Thorax*, 55: 987–99.

WHO (World Health Organization) (2005) *WHO Framework Convention on Tobacco Control*. Geneva: WHO.

Wiltshire, S., Bancroft, A., Amos, A. and Parry, O. (2001) 'They're doing people a service' – qualitative study of smoking, smuggling and social deprivation, *British Medical Journal*, 323: 203–7.

World Bank (2003) *Tobacco Control at a Glance*. Washington, DC: World Bank.

18 Housing, health and wellbeing: a public health action priority

Alex Marsh

This chapter summarizes the wide variety of ways in which housing can influence health and wellbeing. In addition to assessing the links between housing and physical and mental health, the social significance of housing and how this relates to health and quality of life will be given detailed consideration. This will be followed with a brief assessment of the manner in which housing features in public health policy in Britain. Significant arguments throughout the chapter include the central importance of housing to wellbeing, the fundamental importance of securing healthy housing and the need to treat housing as a public health priority.

The long-term relationship between housing and public health

Some of the earliest public health interventions were concerned with the link between poverty, poor housing and disease. Housing conditions for many living in the urban areas that developed rapidly in the wake of the Industrial Revolution were appalling. Governments of mid nineteenth-century Britain felt compelled to respond to the direct effects of poor housing upon health. Poor households in Britain lived in housing that was high density and overcrowded, poorly ventilated and damp, and lacking adequate access to clean water and waste disposal. The mechanisms by which such housing affected health were not necessarily clear, but poor housing was seen to be strongly associated with illnesses such as cholera, tuberculosis and diarrhoea. Pathbreaking interventions such as the Public Health Act 1848 gave public bodies powers over new building, to prevent the unhealthy use of existing houses, to close or demolish individual dwellings that were unfit for human habilitation and to demolish and clear areas of insanitary housing (Holmans 1987).

Wen poor housing and health may have been taken as a spur to an 150 years, and to many it seems self evident, the relationship table. The empirical evidence to demonstrate how housing im- extensive and compelling than might be expected. The same the positive impact of interventions to improve housing condi- 001; Saegert *et al.* 2003). This is in part because disentangling the ealth from the influence of a range of other socioeconomic and contextual variables is a formidable challenge. It is also because the pathways through which housing can influence health and wellbeing are varied and subtle.

Housing and health is an active area of current research, but it is dominated by relatively small studies utilizing diverse methodologies and measures of health. As a consequence, the full picture remains rather obscure. Only occasionally are large scale studies undertaken that interrogate diverse aspects of the relationship between housing and health. A recent example is the World Health Organization (WHO) Regional Office for Europe study to evaluate housing and health in seven European Cities (Bonnefoy *et al.* 2003). Similarly, only a small number of studies are prospective and adopt randomized research designs using control groups (Thomson *et al.* 2001). Consequently, the quality and weight of evidence supporting different aspects of the relationship between housing and health vary. While some are reasonably well established, others are less well supported and their practical significance is questioned. Shaw (2004: 403) nonetheless argues on the basis of the evidence available that housing now affects health in a myriad of relatively minor ways, which together result in housing forming one of the key social determinants of health. While the evidence may be less complete therefore, it is sufficient to mandate a policy concern with the link between housing and health.

The impact of housing on health

The appreciation of the impact of housing upon wellbeing has moved well beyond the concerns of the early public health reformers. In addition to the impact of infectious and chronic disease upon physical health, it is now recognized that housing, viewed not only as the dwelling but also as the immediate physical and social environment, can influence, both directly and indirectly, many dimensions of physical and mental health (Krieger and Higgins 2002; Shaw 2004; Asthana and Halliday 2006) among others. The WHO has recently made public a valuable working document which brings together and assesses the strength of the evidence relating to a substantial number of the potential connections between housing and health (WHO 2006).

The social significance of housing is fundamental. It is a key arena in which social identity is shaped. It is a key mechanism through which individuals and households negotiate the boundary between the public and the private spheres. It is a symbol of social status and a source of social stratification. Recognition of the full significance of housing goes beyond important questions of hygiene and sanitation to trace out impacts of housing upon wellbeing that flow from relative housing positions: the implications of experiencing particular housing circumstances become fundamentally contextual. Furthermore, the link between housing and health needs to be viewed from the perspective of the life course. It is important to understand both the way in which risks experienced at different ages combine to increase risk of disease and also that wellbeing is influenced by more than current housing circumstances alone. Even if housing circumstances in adulthood are satisfactory an exposure to poor housing conditions in the early years can lead to a lower level of health and wellbeing in adulthood (Marsh *et al.* 1999). In this sense, housing history matters.

Impact of housing on physical health

The health concerns with housing began with the impact on physical wellbeing. The relationship between housing and physical health continues to be an active research field, but the areas of interest have broadened. Research has provided evidence of the impact of physical and biological aspects of housing upon health and has identified accessibility and accidents as further areas of concern.

Physical aspects of housing

The main physical aspects of housing that have been investigated for their potentially negative impact upon health are dampness and mould, extremes of temperature (both hot and cold), overcrowding, indoor air quality and the use of problematic construction materials such as lead or asbestos.

Dampness and mould growth have been associated with a wide range of ailments including respiratory disease, eczema, asthma and rhinitis. Extremes of temperature have been clearly identified as a risk factor in excess deaths either in winter or summer, with older people being particularly at risk. Poor indoor air quality can result from a number of sources including inadequate ventilation or location near a major source of pollution such as a main road. It can also be associated with the behaviours and activities of the inhabitants such as smoking or the use of cleaning materials or paints that include irritants or volatile organic compounds. Poor indoor air quality can be linked to respiratory diseases such as asthma. A further risk associated with location is the presence of radon gas, which occurs naturally in higher concentrations in some areas and is linked to an increased risk of lung cancer. The use of lead in the residential context, in water pipes or paint, or in indoor air as a consequence of burning lead based fuels, is problematic because it has been shown to increase the risk of neurological and behavioural problems and impaired cognitive abilities in children. It has also been identified as having a range of adverse impacts on adults, including anaemia, gastrointestinal effects and impaired reproductive health. Asbestos was a popular construction material before it was clearly linked to certain types of lung disease and cancer. It is still present in some buildings constructed in the early Second World War period. There is also some evidence that living for extended periods in neighbourhoods subject to significant traffic noise increases the risk of heart attacks, emphasizing the need to consider housing as comprising features beyond the dwelling itself.

Many of these features of housing have been analysed in isolation. However, it is clear that there are interconnections between many of them. Dampness and mould, for example, may be a product of poor construction methods, but can also be associated with inappropriate indoor temperatures and as a consequence of inadequate ventilation and heating systems. The intersection of these problems increases exposure and the risk of an injury to health.

Biological aspects of housing

Rodents such as rats and mice, including the parasites they harbour, pests such as cockroaches, house dust mites and cats and dogs can all plausibly be argued to represent risk factors in disease. In most cases the risk is related to allergies and increased sensitivities or to respiratory problems. Asthma is a major concern.

However, there is rather less solid evidence available regarding the impact of biological aspects of housing upon health. The evidence for disease attributed to rats, mice or parasites is relatively limited, although this is as much because it has not been extensively researched as because it has been identified not to be an issue. Dust mite allergies are reasonably well established, but their occurrence in numbers sufficient to trigger allergic reaction requires more specific indoor hygrothermal conditions, sufficiently high temperature and moisture levels than is commonly recognized (WHO 2006). This means that modern dwellings with central heating can be a more favourable habitat for house dust mites than older, draughtier and colder dwellings. The impact of exposure to cats and dogs has a more mixed impact upon wellbeing, but there is some evidence that significant exposure to cats in childhood can increase the chances of allergic reaction.

Accessibility

While some people are born with physical impairments or develop an impairment in early life, ageing brings some degree of physical impairment to many people. This in turn raises the question of the design of dwellings and the negative impact of inappropriate design upon wellbeing. Poor accessibility is associated with poor subjective wellbeing.

Accessibility relates to both external access to the property and internal layout and design. Features such as steep steps to the front door can present problems for those with mobility problems. A raised sill at the foot of a front door can be a sufficient barrier effectively to trap someone with serious mobility problems in their own home. Poor exterior access can therefore lead to reduced social participation. Poor internal layout such as narrow doorways or awkward angles between doors can result in inhabitants such as wheelchair users not being able to make use of all the rooms in their dwelling. More generally, insufficient space in rooms and hallways reduces the flexibility with which the dwelling can be used and its accessibility for those with mobility problems. Standard features such as high sided baths or shower trays can represent major barriers to those with physical impairments. This can result in poor standards of hygiene, which not only raise potential health issues but also can further impede social participation through conscious withdrawal from social contact.

While people with physical impairments may choose to move to a property having appraised its suitability, those with progressive impairments may find themselves living in properties that are becoming less accessible over time. This is often the case with older people who remain in the family home and find that steps and stairs, low level electrical sockets, standard bathroom equipment and high kitchen cupboards become more difficult to negotiate. One solution to this is to move to different accommodation. But the social significance of home and its intimate connection with wellbeing, discussed further below, should not be neglected in this context. The disruption associated with reloc particularly if it feels forced rather than chosen, can have a considerable negative impact upon wellbeing.

Over the last decade it has become routine to talk about the need to design lifetime homes. These are dwellings that are flexible and accessible to occupants of all ages and degrees of mobility. Aspirations to achieve such dwellings are embodied in English building regulations. However, the construction industry in Britain is a long way from embedding true accessibility in the design of all new residential property. In part this is because of issues of demand. The accessibility of the dwelling to those with mobility problems is not an issue for most households buying new properties and there is a question of affordability. Building dwellings that are bigger and more flexible typically means building more expensive dwellings in a country where house prices are already high relative to incomes.

Accidents

A fourth physical dimension of housing that can impact upon wellbeing is the exposure of occupants to the risk of accidents. This is not just a question of design but also of behaviour and utilization. Stairs and balconies may not represent a significant risk of falls for a household of adults without physical impairments but become a risk factor for the young and, particularly in the case of stairs, the old. Poor design such as insufficient kitchen workspace, poor lighting or insufficient storage facilities for hazardous materials such as cleaning products can increase the risk of accidents. The risk is also increased by loose fittings such as carpets or rugs. Gas and electricity supplies and heating systems, particularly fires and fireplaces, represent a source of accident risk. But risks arising from physical features of the dwelling can be compounded by utilization of the dwelling. In particular, overcrowding is associated with an increased risk of accident. The recent WHO LARES pan European study also identified an association between sleep disturbance and accidents. Some 22 per cent of those reporting an accident when responding to the survey also reported that their sleep had been disturbed during the previous four weeks (WHO 2004). This is not an association that had previously been explored in the literature.

Mental health

The link between housing and mental health has received limited attention when compared with the research effort directed at exploring the links between housing and physical health. There has been some interest in investigating the direct impact of the presen   c compounds within the home upon neurological problems, but more
                 ncern is with the link between housing circumstances and poor mental
                 ally (see Evans *et al.* 2003 for a recent review).
              research has focused upon the question of the way in which specific
              ics can be a cause of depression or anxiety. There is evidence that
              n increase the likelihood of suffering from depression, particularly
              en (Smith *et al.* 1993). Other negative housing characteristics such
              noise levels, particularly if originating outside the dwelling, have

also been identified as associated with a greater likelihood of poor mental health. Sleep disruption or deprivation, which may be a consequence of these negative types of housing characteristics, are also associated with poorer mental health.

Another branch of research examines poor housing conditions more generally. This can encompass a concern with the state of structural repair, an absence of amenities (such as running water), or temperature control inappropriate or inadequate for local climatic conditions. An association between poor conditions and the likelihood of poorer mental health is reasonably well established. Poor housing conditions have also been associated with broader problems such as poorer adjustment to participation in education and reduced educational performance.

Affordability

An aspect of housing that has attracted increasing research attention has less to do with the physical characteristics of a dwelling and more to do with the costs associated with maintaining occupancy. The affordability or otherwise of a dwelling can affect both physical and mental health, directly and indirectly.

If lower-income households have to spend a large proportion of their income on housing because that is all that is available locally then, if they keep up to date with their housing payments, this reduces the amount of money available for other necessities. One consequence of this may be economizing on fuel and heating. Other consequences may be economizing on food or reducing social participation. Any of these consequences can have negative implications for wellbeing. While this might be thought of as simply a question of poverty, it is clear that housing policy has the potential to mediate the link between low-income and poor housing. For much of its history one of the objectives of council housing in Britain was to provide housing at rents below market levels so that lower-income households could occupy properties of a better quality than those they could afford on the market.

If, on the other hand, households are not able to keep up with their housing payments then this can be a source of stress and depression. In the late 1990s attention was directed at mortgage arrears and mortgage possession as a psychosocial determinant of health (Nettleton and Burrows 1998, 2000). This literature demonstrates that not only are the health consequences of insecure housing significant, they can potentially affect a wide range of households beyond low-income households living in poor-quality rented accommodation.

The social significance of housing

Some sociologists think of the home as a key source of ontological security (Saunders 1990; Dupuis and Thorns 1998), which is defined by Giddens (1991) as the confidence that most human beings have in the continuity of their self identity and in the constancy of their social and material environment. Ontological security is hypothesized as integral to a sense of wellbeing. Hence, disruption or challenge to this sense of security can impact negatively upon wellbeing. This is part of the explanation for why issues such as mortgage arrears or repossessions should be a health concern. Mortgage repossession can be a source of stress, shame and embarrassment because it carries implications for social standing. In a society in which home ownership is the norm, losing one's home might be interpreted as having failed as a citizen.

The recent interest in housing as a psychosocial determinant of health goes beyond the important question of mortgage arrears and possessions. Increasingly there is a concern to understand the way that the diverse social roles played by housing impact upon health. In particular, the importance of housing as a sanctuary and a sphere in which control and freedom can be exercised has been recognized in the context of wellbeing and mental health. Those who do not perceive their dwelling as a private space over which they can exercise control are likely to report poorer mental health. Single-person households can derive greater benefits from this sense of control over the private domain than multi-person households (Kearns *et al.* 2000). One of the sharpest illustrations of the policy significance of recognizing the meaning of home to its occupants is provided by the literature on housing adaptations. Heywood (2005) provides a valuable discussion of the impact of adaptations to assist households with impairments with daily living. Insensitive major adaptations, such as the installation of through lifts between floors, that households feel have been imposed upon them through a process they cannot control, can be perceived as so intrusive that any benefit from the adaptation is undermined by the way it disrupts the household's sense that the dwelling is their own home, which in turn has a negative impact upon their wellbeing.

Housing circumstances are a key signal of social status. A desirable address adds to one's social standing, whereas having a certain postcode can result in being subject to negative perceptions, labelling and discrimination. Housing location can therefore affect life chances directly through access to amenities, services and schools or employment. Living in a poor-quality neighbourhood can result in fear of crime, which has a direct impact upon mental health and a further direct negative effect upon physical health if it results in reduced activity levels and social participation, because people prefer safety by remaining behind closed doors (see Chapter 6 on social exclusion for further insights). Neighbourhood can also affect wellbeing more indirectly through the stigma attached to living in particular localities. The ghettoization of particular locations can impact negatively upon residents' perceptions of themselves.

Although more work is required, there is also some evidence that those who experience relatively poor housing conditions in areas of generally good housing are likely to experience more negative feelings about their health than those experiencing similar conditions in areas of relatively poor housing (Ghodsian and Fogelman 1988).

This finding resonates with the debates that have followed Wilkinson's (1996) argument about the importance of relativities in social position in determining health outcomes (see Chapter 4 for a full discussion of social positioning).

Homelessness and health

The association between rooflessness or rough sleeping and physical and mental health is well established. Roofless households are at greater risk of a range of chronic and infectious diseases, a wide range of mental health problems, and of engaging in risky behaviours involving the misuse of alcohol and illegal drugs. Homeless households are also less likely to be able to access health services. Questions of causation continue to be debated. Does homelessness cause health problems or is it those with health problems who are more likely to find themselves homeless (Johnson *et al.* 1997; Kemp *et al.* 2006)? There is evidence that movement into settled accommodation can reduce risk behaviours that are of central concern to public health. Aidala *et al.* (2005) identify a significant reduction in risks of drug use, needle use, needle sharing and unprotected sex among their sample of homeless households who moved into stable housing compared to those who remained homeless.

In the UK context homelessness refers to a range of insecure housing circumstances short of absolute rooflessness. This can include hostel accommodation, bed and breakfast hotels, or sleeping on a friend's sofa. Living in various forms of temporary accommodation can impact negatively upon health through, for example, inadequate access to appropriate food storage and preparation facilities. It can also impact upon educational achievement if families need to relocate repeatedly. Given the social status attached to housing, an absence of settled accommodation can also impact directly on wellbeing through both its stigmatizing effects and the lack of control and autonomy in the private sphere (Dunn 2002). Hence, less severe types of homelessness represent both a risk to health in the short term and can contribute over the longer term to social inequalities and the consequent inequalities in health.

Taking a holistic perspective

The recent interest in housing as a psychosocial determinant of health has highlighted the importance of a variety of aspects of housing upon mental health and subjective wellbeing. However, the significance of the issue becomes greater once it is set within the context of arguments about the need to move away from a rigid separation between physical and mental health and recognize the interactions between the two. Through its impact upon key physical systems, poor mental health can in the longer term lead to less good physical health. It can also lead to consequences for physical health in the short term (Whooley *et al.* 1999).

The issue is, however, more complex. If housing acts as a signal of social status and at the same time housing trajectories matter, then this opens up the further possibility that the way in which given housing circumstances impact upon health will differ between households. Crudely, does a particular dwelling represent a step up or a step down the housing, and therefore social, ladder? Moving from being homeless to renting a flat in the social rented sector may represent a step up, resulting in improved physical and mental health. In contrast, finding oneself in the same flat as the result of having one's owner occupied dwelling repossessed can have a negative impact upon wellbeing.

It is also important to recognize that housing circumstances interact with other health risks and resources in diverse ways (Smith *et al.* 2003). For example, an involuntary move from owner occupation to renting as a result of mortgage repossession may impact negatively upon health, while leaving owner occupation for renting as a means of escaping domestic violence may mean that poorer housing circumstances are associated with an improvement in physical and mental health. In the latter case, physical housing circumstances may not be as good, but housing is once again fulfilling its role as a place of privacy and safety over which control can be exercised. Such a move can also give access to new resources for social support that can increase resilience in the face of stresses and health risks. This type of complexity means that the scope for identifying strong direct relationships between particular types of housing condition and specific health problems will always be constrained. It has led to calls for a more holistic, social ecological understanding of the relationship between housing and health and the need for multi-level evaluation strategies (Allen 2000; Hartig *et al.* 2003; Saegert *et al.* 2003).

Housing and health policy

The Acheson report (DoH 1998) highlighted housing and environment as areas which policy needed to address if health inequalities were to be reduced. Under the current Labour administration policy statements have explicitly recognized the wider social determinants of health, and within that the role of housing. The NHS Plan (DoH 2000) articulates ten core principles to underpin the modernization of the NHS. One of these relates to tackling health inequalities and preventing ill health. It includes the re-cognition that housing is one of the social, environmental and economic factors upon which good health depends. This agenda is taken forward through *Tackling Health Inequalities: A Programme for Action* (DoH 2003). References to housing occur throughout the document. The focus is primarily upon improving housing conditions, particularly for children; developing more effective strategies to prevent and address homelessness at local level; and addressing fuel poverty among vulnerable groups. The monitoring of this programme of action includes the number of homeless families with children living in temporary accommodation and the proportion of households living in non-decent housing among its national headline indicators. In the government's terms a decent home is one that is warm, weatherproof and has reasonably modern facilities. The requirements, while important, are therefore relatively modest. If all dwellings were to meet the Decent Homes Standard this would not necessarily mean that all the aspects of housing that can impact negatively upon wellbeing would have been addressed.

The first status report on the programme for action was able to highlight a significant reduction in the proportion of households in England living in non decent accom-modation, from 44 per cent in 1996 to 30 per cent in 2003. It also reported significant progress in reducing fuel poverty, but a mixed picture regarding homelessness. While the number of families with children living in bed and breakfast accommodation, usually considered the most unsuitable, had decreased, the number living in other types of temporary accommodation had increased (DoH 2005). These positive messages need to be seen in the context of the broader question of housing supply. It is widely accepted that the current rate of house building in Britain is falling well short of the number of households that wish to live independently (Barker 2004). The result is that house prices are higher than they otherwise would be and there are higher levels of delayed household formation, involuntary sharing or hidden homelessness. This is arguably as significant for wellbeing, if less immediately apparent, as the issues that policy is targeting. Housing specialists continue to debate whether the steps the government has taken to address this problem through increased housing supply are adequate.

One of the key features of the current government's approach is a strong emphasis upon the need to draw on expertise from a range of fields and for cross departmental working at both national and local level to address inequalities effectively. Collaborations at a strategic level such as Health Improvement Programmes (HimPs) or on more specific topics such as achieving positive outcomes on health and homelessness are embodied in the approach taken by the Office of Deputy Prime Minister/Department of Health (ODPM/DoH 2004). However, it is important to recognize that while positive examples of collaboration can be identified (see Chapter 16 for examples of this), the difficulties of working across sectors on health and housing issues should not be underestimated (Harrison and Heywood 2000).

Providing healthy housing as a public health action priority

Housing can impact upon health in many ways, both direct and indirect, but the available evidence on the relationships is less extensive than is desirable. Similarly, reviews of the evidence on the efficacy of housing interventions in improving health do not point to the compelling conclusion that housing interventions have major positive impacts upon wellbeing. One might conclude therefore that this is not a priority area for action. However, this would be a mistake. First, many past policy interventions have tended to be too narrowly focused to make major impacts upon health. In this regard, some of the current government's initiatives involving more broad based area renewal may have more chance of succeeding. Second, evaluation strategies have not always been sufficiently sophisticated to be able to isolate the impact of changes in housing circumstances. The very complexity of the links between housing and health, alongside the fact that poor housing is often associated with a range of other health risk factors, means that it will be a long time before the weight of evidence is sufficient to convince the hardened sceptic.

Yet, with the psychosocial dimensions to this relationship only recently beginning to be explored, the richness of the connection between home and wellbeing is becoming increasingly apparent. Healthy housing is a fundamental building block for both personal identity and social participation. It shapes quality of life and life chances. As such it is fundamental to human wellbeing and health inequalities. What is required now is research and policy informed by this more subtle appreciation of the interaction between housing, broader socioeconomic risk factors and wellbeing. A concern with the housing circumstances of the population most certainly warrants a place at the centre of public health concerns.

References

Aidala, A., Cross, J.E., Stall, R., Harre, D. and Sumartojo, E. (2005) Housing status and HIV risk behaviors: implications for prevention and policy, *Aids and Behavior*, 9(3): 251–65.

Allen, C. (2000) On the 'physiological dope' problematic in housing and illness research: towards a critical realism of housing and health, *Housing, Theory and Society*, 17(1): 49–67.

Asthana, S. and Halliday, J. (2006) *What Works in Tackling Health Inequalities? Pathways, Policies and Practice through the Lifecourse*. Bristol: The Policy Press.

Barker, K. (2004) *Review of Housing Supply: Delivering Stability – Securing our Future Housing Needs*. London: HM Treasury.

Bonnefoy, X., Matthias, B., Moissonnier, B., Monolbaev, K. and Robbel, N. (2003) Housing and health in Europe: preliminary results of a pan-European study, *American Journal of Public Health*, 93(9): 1559–63.

DoH (Department of Health) (1998) *Inequalities in Health: Report of an Independent Inquiry Chaired by Sir Donald Acheson*. London: The Stationery Office.

DoH (Department of Health) (2000) *The NHS Plan: A Plan for Investment, a Plan for Reform*. Cm 4818-1. London: The Stationery Office.

DoH (Department of Health) (2003) *Tackling Health Inequalities: A Programme for Action*. London: Department of Health.

DoH (Department of Health) (2005) *Tackling Health Inequalities: Status Report on the Programme for Action*. London: Department of Health.

Dunn, J.R. (2002) Housing and inequalities in health: a study of socioeconomic dimensions of housing and self reported health from a survey of Vancouver residents, *Journal of Epidemiology and Community Health*, 56(9): 671–81.

Dupuis, A. and Thorns, D. (1998) Home, home ownership and the search for ontological security, *Sociological Review*, 46(1): 24–47.

Evans, G., Wells, N. and Moch, A. (2003) Housing and mental health: a review of the evidence and a methodological and conceptual critique, *Journal of Social Issues*, 59(3): 475–500.

Ghodsian, M. and Fogelman, K. (1988) *A Longitudinal Study of Housing Circumstances in Childhood and Early Adulthood*. NCDS User Support Group Working Paper 29. London: City University.

Giddens, A. (1991) *Modernity and Self-identity: Self and Society in the Late Modern Age*. Cambridge: Polity Press.

Harrison, L. and Heywood, F. (2000) *Health Begins at Home: Planning at the Health–housing Interface for Older People*. Bristol: The Policy Press.

Hartig, T., Johansson, G. and Kylin, C. (2003) Residence in the social ecology of stress and restoration, *Journal of Social Issues*, 59(3): 611–36.

Heywood, F. (2005) Adaptation: altering the house to restore the home, *Housing Studies*, 20(4): 531–47.

Holmans, A. (1987) *Housing Policy in Britain*. London: Croom Helm.

Johnson, T.P., Freels, S.A., Parsons, J.A. and Vangeest, J.B. (1997) Substance abuse and homelessness: social selection or social adaptation? *Addiction*, 92(4): 437–45.

Kearns, A., Hiscock, R., Ellaway, A. and Macintyre, S. (2000) 'Beyond four walls': the psychosocial benefits of home: evidence from West Central Scotland, *Housing Studies*, 15(3): 387–410.

Kemp, P.A., Neale, J. and Robertson, M. (2006) Homelessness among problem drug users: prevalence, risk factors and trigger events, *Health & Social Care in the Community*, 14(4): 319–28.

Krieger, J. and Higgins, D. (2002) Housing and health: time again for public health action, *American Journal of Public Health*, 92(5): 758–68.

Marsh, A., Gordon, D., Pantazis, C. and Heslop, P. (1999) *Home Sweet Home? The Impact of Poor Housing on Health*. Bristol: The Policy Press.

Nettleton, S. and Burrows, R. (1998) Mortgage debt, insecure home ownership and health: an exploratory analysis, in M. Bartley, D. Blane and G. Davey-Smith (eds) *The Sociology of Health Inequality*. Oxford: Blackwell.

Nettleton, S. and Burrows, R. (2000) When a capital investment becomes an emotional loss: the health consequences of the experience of mortgage repossession in England, *Housing Studies*, 15(3): 463–79.

ODPM/DoH (Office of Deputy Prime Minister/Department of Health) (2004) *Achieving Positive Shared Outcomes in Health and Homelessness: A Homelessness and Housing Support Directorate Advice Note to Local Authorities, Primary Care Trusts and Other Partners*. London: ODPM.

Saegert, S., Klitzman, S., Freudenberg, N., Cooperman-Mroczek, J. and Nassar, S. (2003) Healthy housing: a structured review of published evaluations of US interventions to improve health by modifying housing in the United States, 1990–2001, *American Journal of Public Health*, 93(9): 1471–77.

Saunders, P. (1990) *A Nation of Home Owners*. London: Unwin Hyman.

Shaw, M. (2004) Housing and public health, *Annual Review of Public Health*, 25: 397–418.

Smith, C., Kearns, R. and Abbott, M. (1993) Housing stressors, social support and psychological distress, *Social Science and Medicine*, 37: 603–12.

Smith, S., Easterlow, D., Munro, M. and Turner, K. (2003) Housing as health capital: how health trajectories and housing paths are linked, *Journal of Social Issues*, 59(3): 501–25.

Thomson, H., Petticrew, M. and Morrison, D. (2001) Health effects of housing improvements: systematic review of intervention studies, *British Medical Journal*, 323: 187–90.

WHO (2004) *Review of Evidence on Housing and Health*. Background document to Fourth Ministerial Conference on Environment and Health, Budapest, 23–25 June. Copenhagen: WHO Regional Office for Europe.

WHO (2006) *Report on the WHO Technical Meeting on Quantifying Disease from Inadequate Housing*. Bonn, Germany, 28–30 November 2005. Copenhagen: WHO Regional Office for Europe.

Whooley, M., Kip, K., Cauley, J., Ensrud, K., Nevitt, M. and Browner, W. (1999) Depression, falls and risk of fracture in older women, *Archives of Internal Medicine*, 159: 484–90.

Wilkinson, R. (1996) *Unhealthy Societies: The Afflictions of Inequality*. London: Routledge.

Author Index

Subject Index